Nursing Education in the AI Era

Delaney Wright La Rosa
Danica Fulbright Sumpter
Sally Carlisle • Kenya V. Beard
Editors

Nursing Education in the AI Era

Practical Guidance for Educators to Advance Equitable Care

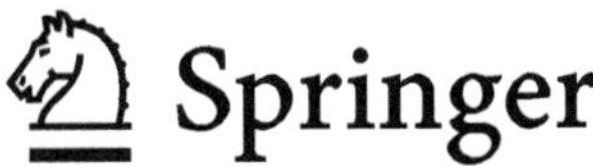

Springer

Editors
Delaney Wright La Rosa (iD)
Florida State University College of Nursing
Tallahassee, FL, USA

Danica Fulbright Sumpter
CS Innovations
Round Rock, TX, USA

Sally Carlisle
Nursing
Mercy University
Bradenton, FL, USA

Kenya V. Beard
Mercy University
Dobbs Ferry, NY, USA

ISBN 978-3-032-12401-2   ISBN 978-3-032-12402-9   (eBook)
https://doi.org/10.1007/978-3-032-12402-9

This Springer imprint is published by the registered company Springer Nature Switzerland AG
The registered company address is: Gewerbestrasse 11, 6330 Cham, Switzerland

If disposing of this product, please recycle the paper.

Foreword

I still see the spreadsheets—color-coded, desperate, hopeful.

My grandfather was in his late 1980s when the sundowning began. As darkness fell each evening, so did his clarity, his calm, his connection to the world he'd known. Our family—accomplished professionals, problem-solvers by trade—found ourselves reduced to amateur caregivers, armed with nothing but lists and love. We tracked medications in columns, documented behaviors in rows, trying to impose order on the chaos of a mind unwinding.

The system that was supposedly built on dignity and grace? It offered us neither. No guidance. No support. Just forms to fill and bills to pay.

The homecare and hospital visits were brutal. My grandfather, confused and frightened, sat in sterile rooms surrounded by beeping machines he couldn't understand. Staff, depending on the shift and stress level, reduced him to a room number, a diagnosis code. Except for the nurses. The quarterbacks of the healthcare system. They were the only human faces in an inhuman design. Somehow, amid the impossible churn of their schedules, they'd pause—to touch his shoulder, to speak his name, to see the husband and father still flickering behind the fog. For someone who had contributed meaningfully to his family, his community, and to the very system now failing him, you would think dignity would be a built-in feature of care. It wasn't.

When he finally passed at 92, after years of slow disappearance, I found myself asking: This is healthcare? This is how we honor our elders? We invest in this system with every paycheck—where was the intelligence, artificial or otherwise, to help us find our way? Where was the support that could have predicted the crisis points, connected us to resources, or simply given those nurses more time to be present?

Years later. Different hospital. Different crisis. Same revelation.

My wife had been in labor for so long that time lost all meaning. Our oldest child seemed determined to arrive on his own timeline. The medical team offered vague reassurances. The monitors sang their incomprehensible songs. We were young, terrified, and dependent on a system that felt more like machinery than medicine. As complications mounted, so did uncertainty. Everyone moved carefully within a system that constrained healer and patient alike.

But then there was our night nurse.

She never really left us. Even when caring for others, we felt held by her presence. She checked on my wife constantly—not just the clinical checks, but the human ones. A cool cloth. A repositioned pillow. A quiet word when despair crept in.

And she charted. Every detail, every shift in tone or expression. I watched her document with the precision of someone who knew these weren't just notes—they were a story she was writing for whoever would need to read it next.

When our son finally arrived, he took one enormous gasp—and both his lungs collapsed. Complete pneumothorax. In that moment of supposed joy, we plunged into terror.

But our nurse had already summoned the surgeons. Her vigilant charting, her clinical intuition, her refusal to dismiss a subtle concern—she'd seen what the machines hadn't. The team performed a double thoracostomy, inserting tiny chest tubes to save a tiny life.

My son breathed. We breathed. The nurse smiled—the quiet smile of someone who had just done what she was trained to do, not knowing she had done something miraculous.

At the time, I was a young clinician focused on fertility and labor. But I learned more about vigilance, intuition, and presence that night than I had in years of training. The most powerful technology in that room wasn't the device or the monitor. It was a nurse who knew how to pay attention—to both the data and the human beneath it.

These two experiences—years apart, but united by truth—taught me everything I needed to know about the future of healthcare. In both cases, nurses were the bridge between human need and systemic failure. They preserved dignity when the system forgot it. They noticed what the protocols didn't.

Now, as we stand at the edge of healthcare's AI transformation, I think about those nurses constantly. What if my grandfather's care team had access to AI tools that lifted the burden of documentation, allowing them more time for touch and presence? What if predictive models could have flagged the warning signs of his decline and routed us toward support—before we were left with nothing but spreadsheets and panic?

What if that labor nurse had been supported by AI-enhanced monitoring that validated her instincts? What if her intuition had been amplified rather than left to stand alone?

But here's the essential point: in both cases, technology would have only mattered if it served the human connection. My grandfather didn't need an algorithm. He needed someone who still saw him. My son didn't just need clinical precision. He needed someone who could read between the lines of the data to sense danger before it struck.

These stories reveal not professional failure but systemic constraint. Every caregiver—physician, technician, aide—was trapped in the same web of protocols that trapped us as patients. But nurses, standing at the intersection of data and humanity, monitoring and meaning, somehow kept finding ways to bridge what the system had severed.

The Choice Before Us

We're not just integrating tools. We're deciding what nursing will mean in an age when machines can mimic judgment, predict outcomes, and summarize lives in a paragraph of code.

Will AI free nurses to be more present, like those who comforted my grandfather? Or distance them further from the bedside?

Will it heighten clinical intuition, like the nurse who saved my son? Or replace it with algorithmic certainty that misses the moment?

Will it help build systems that offer dignity and grace to all? Or will it deepen the divide between those with access and those left alone with spreadsheets and hope?

These are not technical questions. They are moral ones. And they demand educators who understand that their role is not merely to teach new tools—but to shape, question, and sometimes resist them in defense of what makes nursing irreplaceable.

A Personal Covenant

I write this foreword as someone who has stood on both sides of the bed rail—as a family member desperate for help, as a clinician trying to give it, and now as someone working to ensure that technology serves humanity, not the other way around.

To the nurse educators reading this: you are preparing students for a world where the line between human and artificial intelligence will blur. Teach them how to navigate that blur without losing themselves. Help them see that their value lies not just in what they know, but in how they choose to show up—in how they presence themselves with suffering.

To the students: learn the tools, master the platforms. But never forget the desperation that families chart in color-coded cells when the system fails them. Never forget that behind every data point is someone's grandfather, someone's child—someone's whole world hanging in the balance.

To all of us: remember that we are not just building smarter systems. We are building the moral terrain in which people will face their most vulnerable moments. And we owe them—deeply, completely—nothing less than technology that amplifies compassion, rather than replacing it.

The Path Forward

This book offers a map for a landscape still being drawn. It insists that every patient matters equally, invites ethical reflection, and refuses to let efficiency eclipse dignity. Most importantly, it makes clear: the future of nursing isn't about choosing between the human and the artificial. It's about learning how to weave them together in service of healing.

As you read, I invite you to carry with you the image of two nurses—one offering dignity to an aging man losing his grip on the world, the other seeing what machines could not in a moment of birth and peril. They are the compass. They are the promise.

The tools will evolve. The challenges will shift. But the core truth remains: at the heart of nursing is something no algorithm can replicate—one human being, fully present to another, in their time of greatest need.

That is the flame this book will help you tend.

That is the future we must build together.

May we choose wisely. May we never forget why we chose this profession. And may every advancement in technology serve to make us more human, not less.

The future is calling. Let's make sure it sounds like hope—

Microsoft, New York City, NY, USA   Michael J. Jabbour

Contents

AI in Healthcare and Education

1

Ashley Graham-Perel

Human intelligence laid the foundation of healthcare advancements, and its extension of artificial intelligence is poised to serve as the catalyst for groundbreaking innovations that redefine the very limits of possibility. Artificial intelligence (AI) has become an integral force at the crossroads of healthcare and education, invariably shaping and reimagining the future of these fields. Since emerging in the 1950s, AI has made extraordinary strides, particularly between the 2000s and 2020s, expanding its presence across industries such as finance, healthcare, and transportation [1]. In this chapter, the history and evolution of AI in healthcare and education are explored. Additionally, the benefits and challenges of AI, with discussions of medical errors, clinical readiness, and equity, are presented. The current frameworks for ethical and practical integration of AI in nursing are discussed.

It could be argued that concerns surrounding AI largely arise from fears that machines might replace humans, disrupt livelihoods, or potentially harm human well-being. Such concerns reflect a broader anxiety about the increasing role of technology in society. However, the original goal of artificial intelligence was not to replace humans but to first replicate human intelligence and then enhance it [2]. In 1952, Alan Turing introduced the "Turing Test," a groundbreaking method for determining whether a machine could demonstrate intelligence indistinguishable from human cognition [3]. Turing's work laid the foundation for the field of AI, proposing that if a machine could convincingly imitate human responses, it could be considered truly intelligent. In 1956, the term "artificial intelligence" was coined by John McCarthy, a pioneering computer scientist at Dartmouth College, who is often referred to as the "father of AI." McCarthy's vision extended beyond simple replication; he sought to create machines capable of simulating complex human reasoning

A. Graham-Perel (✉)
Office of Engagement and Community Affairs, Columbia University School of Nursing, New York, NY, USA
e-mail: ag4122@cumc.columbia.edu

© The Author(s), under exclusive license to Springer Nature Switzerland AG 2026
D. W. La Rosa et al. (eds.), *Nursing Education in the AI Era*,
https://doi.org/10.1007/978-3-032-12402-9_1

1

and decision-making [3]. His work, along with that of others, aimed not just to match human intelligence but to open the door to future advancements in AI that could revolutionize fields ranging from healthcare to education, transforming society in unimaginable ways.

AI is a broad field that includes any mechanisms designed to cultivate the intelligence of humans through technology and machines [3]. The subfields of AI include terms such as Machine Learning (ML), Deep Learning (DL), Natural Language Processing (NLP), and Computer Vision (CV). Kaul et al. (2020) defined machine learning (ML) as the "pattern identification and analysis; machines can improve with experience from provided data sets" [2] p. 808). In other words, with the use of ML, computers learn from the data received and can produce predictions based on the information it receives [4]. An example of ML in nursing education includes algorithms used to develop the communication skills of nursing students through simulation experiences [5].

The building of ML with neural networks that employ computers with the ability to not only learn patterns but to make decisions is known as DL. Breakthroughs in areas such as speech recognition and computer vision using DL can enhance nursing practice. Wangpitipanit, Jiraporn, and Anderson, (2024) stated, "DL contributes to safer medication management and facilitates remote patient monitoring, enabling nurses to intervene promptly. With its capacity for personalized care, DL holds promise for revolutionizing nursing practices, ultimately resulting in improved patient outcomes and healthcare delivery" [6] p.2). Kaul et al. (2020) defined Natural Learning Processing (NLP) as the "process that enables computers to extract data from human languages and make decisions based on that information" (3, p. 808). In nursing, an example of this subset includes the analysis of data, such as nursing documentation or nursing narratives, to identify trends and patterns in patient care and present recommendations for nurses to provide more effective, evidence-based care [7]. When a computer learns information and builds understanding from information such as images or videos, this is known as CV [2]. In healthcare, this subset of AI has been used to improve disease diagnosis for medical images such as ultrasounds and scans [8].

1.1   Nursing's Involvement in AI

AI has significantly transformed the healthcare landscape, redefining the standards of high-quality care, the modalities of care delivery, and patient health outcomes. From diagnostic imaging to clinical implementation, virtually every aspect of healthcare will be influenced by AI [9, 10]. However, despite being the primary end-users of these technologies, the inclusion of nurses during the critical stages of AI development is limited [11, 12]. As the largest sector of the healthcare workforce, nurses occupy a pivotal position to advocate for AI-driven innovations that enhance efficiency while addressing the diverse needs of patient populations [13], yet their involvement in AI development has remained limited for decades. This gap may be largely attributed to deficiencies in nursing education, particularly in foundational digital literacy and informatics competencies. Without proficiency in the technical language and frameworks of AI development, nurses may struggle to effectively contribute to shaping these technologies to align with the realities of clinical nursing practice. The gap in nursing's involvement in AI development has significant implications for both patient care and the nursing profession. Without the direct input of nurses, AI systems may be designed without consideration for the complexities of nursing workflows, leading to inefficiencies, increased workload, and even potential patient safety risks [14, 15]. Many AI-driven tools are created with a physician-centric model [12, 16, 17], overlooking the critical role that nurses play in patient monitoring, clinical decision-making, and care coordination. As a result, these technologies may not fully align with the realities of nursing practice, forcing nurses to adapt to AI rather than AI being designed to support nursing needs. Moreover, the dearth of nursing representation in AI development exacerbates the digital divide within healthcare, reinforcing the perception that AI is a tool for technologists and physicians rather than an integrated component of interdisciplinary care.

To bridge this gap, it is imperative to integrate AI education into nursing curricula, ensuring that nurses develop the necessary digital literacy and informatics competencies to engage in interdisciplinary collaborations with AI developers [18]. By fostering a deeper understanding of data science, machine learning, and ethical AI implementation, nursing professionals can actively participate in shaping AI-driven solutions that align with clinical workflows and patient-centered care. Additionally, healthcare institutions and policymakers must recognize the importance of nursing involvement in AI governance and decision-making, ensuring that technological advancements reflect the complexities of real-world nursing practice. Without such engagement, AI risks being developed in a vacuum, failing to address the nuanced challenges faced by nurses at the bedside and beyond. Therefore, strategic efforts must be made to empower nurses as key stakeholders in AI development, ensuring that these innovations enhance, rather than hinder, the delivery of safe, equitable, and effective healthcare [19].

The outlook of nursing educators must expand during this AI era. It is imperative that AI be incorporated across nursing curricula to prepare future nurses for a technologically augmented practice environment. A suggested practice for educators is to examine selected foundational nursing theories and explore how their application may be reimagined in the context of AI. For example, Patricia Benner's Novice to Expert theory [20], which outlines the stages of progressive development and nursing competence through experiential learning, invites inquiry into how AI might influence or support each stage of professional growth. Can AI tools accelerate skill acquisition or deepen clinical reasoning for novice nurses? Similarly, Madeleine Leininger's Transcultural Nursing Theory [21], which underscores the necessity of cultural considerations in care, prompts reflection on how AI systems (which are often critiqued for embedded biases—as presented later in this chapter) can be used ethically and effectively to enhance students' understanding of diverse patient populations. How might educators use AI to simulate culturally appropriate care scenarios or critique healthcare disparities? Lastly, Hildegard Peplau's Theory of Interpersonal Relations [22], which centered on the therapeutic nurse-patient relationship, challenges educators to consider how AI might support the development of a nurse's interpersonal competencies. What roles can AI-driven simulations or communication tools play in cultivating emotional intelligence, empathy, and therapeutic dialogue? These examples accentuate the critical need for educators to reevaluate pedagogical approaches that align with both enduring theoretical frameworks and emerging technological realities.

1.2 Benefits and Challenges of AI

Over the past several decades, the nursing profession has evolved significantly from its foundational beginnings into a complex, evidence-informed discipline that must continuously adapt to meet the diverse and growing needs of patients. Despite these advancements, a persistent challenge remains: time. Nurses are frequently constrained by time-consuming responsibilities such as documentation and administrative duties, communication across interdisciplinary teams, and the cognitive work of analyzing patient data, which can reduce time spent in direct patient care and, in some cases, negatively impact patient outcomes [23–25]. These demands are mirrored in nursing education, where time limitations also affect teaching, learning, and clinical preparation. As educators work to equip students for the realities of modern practice, integrating tools that address these constraints becomes imperative. AI could present a promising avenue to optimize both clinical and educational processes. Within academic settings, AI has the potential to reduce administrative burdens, enhance simulation fidelity, personalize learning, and foster clinical reasoning, yet its integration is not without complexity. This section of the chapter will explore both the benefits and challenges of incorporating AI into nursing education and practice, with particular attention to its implications for reducing medical errors, supporting clinical readiness among students and practicing nurses, and promoting (or potentially hindering) equity in healthcare delivery and access to learning technologies.

1.3 Nurses' Well-Being Enhanced with AI

The well-being of nurses is a critical component of both nursing education and professional practice. From the outset of their academic journey, nursing students are introduced to the emotional, physical, and cognitive stressors inherent in the profession. These stressors are not confined to the academic setting but often intensify following licensure, as newly credentialed nurses transition into high-demand clinical environments. As such, nursing education must adopt a dual focus: preparing students to navigate a rigorous curriculum while simultaneously equipping them with the skills and resilience necessary to manage the realities of clinical practice. AI offers valuable opportunities to support this dual imperative. In alignment with Domain 10 of the American Association of Colleges of Nursing's (AACN) 2021 Essentials—which emphasizes the promotion of personal well-being, leadership development, and professional resilience [26], AI can serve as an innovative tool to enhance workflow efficiency, reduce cognitive overload, and promote work-life balance [27]. By streamlining routine tasks and improving access to information, AI holds the potential to reduce burnout, empower clinical decision-making, and foster a more sustainable practice environment for both students and nurses. Moreover, by addressing the specific needs of learners and staff, such as improving organizational skills, structuring clinical or didactic workflows, and adapting content delivery to individual learning styles, AI can be incorporated in a manner that meaningfully supports well-being, professional development, and academic success.

1.4   Improving Clinical Decision Making

In the United States, medical errors are a significant concern, with estimates indicating that over 200,000 patient deaths annually may be attributed to such errors [28]. These statistics include errors in nursing decision making. A growing body of research highlights that nurses' clinical decision-making is shaped by a multitude of factors, including patient-specific conditions, unit staffing levels, communication challenges, organizational culture on decision making, situational awareness, and the nurse's level of clinical expertise—ranging from novice to expert, as described by Benner's theoretical framework [20, 29]. Within nursing education, clinical decision-making is explored through diverse theoretical lenses, encompassing both intuitive and experiential models. Despite this, there remains a notable gap in the integration of artificial intelligence (AI) into nursing curricula [30, 31]. Given AI's capacity to support decision-making through access to large datasets, predictive analytics, and automated tools, it is imperative that nurse educators develop competencies in this domain. Such preparation is essential to equip future nurses with the ability to leverage AI in enhancing clinical judgment and improving patient outcomes.

Nursing education must evolve to reflect the growing influence of AI in healthcare. Preparing future nurses involves not only teaching them what AI does, but also how to work with it responsibly, critically, and compassionately in clinical practice [19]. In practice, AI assists nurses by synthesizing vast amounts of information through machine learning and natural language processing, enabling more accurate diagnoses and care planning [32, 33]. To prepare nurses for practice environments increasingly shaped by intelligent systems, educators must introduce students to how AI can be used to support—and not replace—their clinical reasoning [27]. This includes exposure to AI-driven simulations that model complex patient scenarios and learning to interpret AI-generated recommendations within the context of holistic, patient-centered care.

How can nurse educators ensure that graduates are both competent and confident in using AI technologies to enhance their clinical decision-making? One recommendation is to utilize AI to shape how students process the information they are taught. One method to consider is the Socratic method. In their paper *"Critical Thinking: The Development of an Essential Skill for Nursing Students,"*

Papathanasiou, Fradelos, Kakou, and Kourkouta (2014) emphasize that critical thinking fosters key professional behaviors such as integrity, perseverance, curiosity, and confidence in one's clinical reasoning [34]. These cognitive and affective attributes can be cultivated through methods like Socratic questioning, a pedagogical approach widely employed in both medical and nursing education to stimulate reflective thought and analytical dialogue. Socratic questioning has been examined across diverse contexts, ranging from its use in helping individuals recognize disinformation in media to its application in classrooms, clinical settings, and as an effective study strategy [22].

In the context of tutoring, research has explored student perceptions of AI-based versus human support. While many students value the accessibility and nonjudgmental nature of AI tools such as ChatGPT, human tutors remain preferred for their ability to provide personalized guidance and emotional connection [35]. To translate these principles of critical thinking into practice, nurse educators can integrate emerging tools like generative AI into their teaching strategies to foster critical thinking and clinical judgment. For instance, in a classroom utilizing AI platforms such as ChatGPT, educators might assign students the task of crafting a well-structured prompt related to a clinical scenario or concept. After generating a response from the AI, the focus should shift from passive consumption to active analysis. Through guided Socratic questioning, educators can prompt students to evaluate the AI's output critically. Questions such as, "Is the information provided accurate?", "Does it align with current clinical guidelines?", "What assumptions underlie the AI's response?", and "Are the sources reliable?" can lead to deeper reflection. This method not only mirrors real-world clinical decision-making, where nurses must assess, question, and synthesize information, but also helps students recognize the role of AI as a tool that supports, rather than replaces, their clinical reasoning. By embedding these reflective exercises into the curriculum, nurse educators can cultivate essential habits of mind (such as curiosity, discernment, and analytical rigor) that are foundational to safe and effective nursing practice.

1.5 Classroom Assessment Technique: AI-enhanced Clinical Reasoning Check

1.6 Purpose

To assess students' ability to critically evaluate clinical information using AI as a thinking partner.

Procedure

1. *Prompt Generation (3–5 min):*
   Instruct students to write a short, clinically relevant question or scenario (e.g., "What are the early signs of sepsis in older adults?").
2. *AI Response Review (5 min):*
   Using ChatGPT or a similar tool, students input their prompt and receive a response.
3. *Socratic Evaluation (5–7 min):*
   Individually or in small groups, students answer these guiding questions:

   - Is this information accurate and up to date?
   - What assumptions does the AI make?
   - Is anything important missing?
   - How would you verify the response?

4. *Feedback Collection (2–3 min):*
   Students write a brief reflection or submit a response card:
   - One thing I learned or realized...
   - One question I still have...

Use for Instructors

This Classroom Assessment Technique helps gauge how well students are applying critical thinking and clinical judgment and provides insight into their ability to work with emerging technologies.

1.7   Bias, Ethics, and Equity

Ethical and equity considerations must remain at the forefront of AI integration into healthcare and nursing education [36]. One of the most critical concerns is the propensity of AI technologies to reflect and potentially exacerbate existing societal biases. One of the primary roles nurse educators can undertake is the integration of these concepts into nursing curricula, particularly as they relate to AI applications. This includes teaching students how AI systems are developed, the role of data in shaping algorithmic outputs, and how biases in training data can lead to discriminatory clinical outcomes. Given that structural racism and systemic inequities profoundly shape health outcomes, socioeconomic status, and overall well-being [37, 38], it is imperative that nursing education actively addresses and works to prevent the perpetuation of these injustices through the adoption and application of AI tools.

AI systems are inherently shaped by the data on which they are trained data that are often curated, labeled, and influenced by human judgment. Consequently, these systems inherit and operatively implement the limitations and biases embedded within those datasets. In healthcare, this has already resulted in biased clinical decision-making tools that adversely affect risk assessments, access to care, and treatment recommendations [39]. For example, a pivotal 2019 study demonstrated that an AI-based population health management tool, which used healthcare costs as a proxy for medical need, systematically underestimated the healthcare needs of Black patients compared to their White counterparts, leading to unequal resource allocation [40]. Through the use of evidence-based case studies and current research, educators can illuminate the real-world inequitable consequences of AI implementation and foster critical reflection among students.

Understanding the limitations and assumptions embedded in datasets is crucial for evaluating AI tools used in clinical settings. Educators should empower students to question how data is collected, labeled, and interpreted and to identify potential sources of systemic bias, particularly those rooted in race, socioeconomic status, or other social determinants of health. This kind of analytical training prepares students to assess AI-supported decision-making tools critically and ethically, rather than adopting them uncritically. Numerous clinical algorithms that incorporate race and ethnicity have been shown to produce harmful outcomes for communities of color [41]. Notably, tools such as the American Heart Association's "Get with the Guidelines–Heart Failure Risk Score," the estimated glomerular filtration rate (eGFR), and the Vaginal Birth After Cesarean (VBAC) calculator have demonstrated embedded racial biases, yet continue to be used in clinical settings [42]. These examples underscore the need for critical scrutiny and reform of race-based metrics in healthcare. Nursing education must incorporate the evaluation of race-based clinical algorithms and foster an environment in which students feel empowered to challenge outdated or harmful practices.

The World Health Organization (WHO), in its 2021 report Ethics and Governance of Artificial Intelligence for Health: WHO Guidance, emphasized the global responsibility to develop and regulate AI technologies in a manner that upholds ethical standards and safeguards public health [43]. For nursing education and practice, this necessitates a pedagogical and leadership approach that not only integrates AI competencies but also prioritizes equity, transparency, and accountability in the deployment of AI-driven technologies. Creating inclusive learning environments that support open dialogue on race, equity, and emerging technologies can help students develop the critical consciousness necessary to confront structural inequities in healthcare. By fostering a culture of inquiry, reflection, and action, nursing education can produce practitioners who are not only clinically competent but also committed to advancing social justice through ethical innovation.

Leadership development is another essential component of nursing education that must evolve to address the challenges posed by AI. Nurse educators should cultivate leadership skills that include ethical reasoning, health policy advocacy, and interdisciplinary collaboration. As future leaders in healthcare, nurses must be equipped not only to use AI technologies but also to participate in their ethical design and implementation. Collaborating with data scientists, health informaticists, and policymakers, nurses can advocate for inclusive AI systems that reflect the diversity and complexity of patient populations.

Ethical considerations extend to the core of nursing's professional identity, which is rooted in compassion, empathy, and human connection. While AI can simulate decision-making and even natural language responses, it cannot embody the relational and moral dimensions of nursing practice [44]. The emergence of AI technologies being referred to as "nurses" has raised alarms in regulatory and legislative spaces. States have begun developing laws to protect the professional title of "nurse," affirming that a nurse must be a licensed human being [45]. These legal measures reflect broader concerns about the erosion of trust and the dehumanization of care, as AI begins to take on roles that were once considered exclusively human.

Data privacy, informed consent, and confidentiality are also critical ethical issues that must be addressed as AI tools are implemented in both clinical and educational settings. The use of large-scale health data to train AI systems raises significant questions under the Health Insurance Portability and Accountability Act (HIPAA). While AI tools may analyze de-identified data, re-identification risks remain, particularly when data are combined from multiple sources. Moreover, patients and students may not fully understand how their information is being used, complicating the ethical obligation to obtain informed consent. In the educational realm, AI may assist with adaptive learning suited for individualized student needs [46]. This will require student data and may violate the areas of the Family Educational Rights and Privacy Act (FERPA), which protects the privacy of student education records. In an age where data are both currency and vulnerability, protecting individual rights must be a cornerstone of AI integration in nursing.

To ensure that nursing professionals are prepared to lead ethically in an AI-driven future, nursing education must incorporate robust content on the social, legal, and policy implications of artificial intelligence. This includes teaching students how to critically appraise AI tools, advocate for inclusive algorithm development, and participate in policy creation that governs AI use in healthcare. Without such preparation, nurses may become passive users of tools they do not fully understand, rather than active participants in shaping how technology supports equitable and ethical care. Equity-driven pedagogy should include an understanding of possible inequities in access to AI tools that may widen the digital divide, disproportionately affecting learners in under-resourced settings. Ultimately, embedding ethics and equity into AI education is essential to preserving the core values of nursing while embracing innovation. In support of these concerns, the American Nurses Association's 2022 statement on AI use in nursing advocates for embedding ethical principles, equity, and the profession's core values into AI implementation. It highlights the importance of involving nurses in shaping AI tools to ensure they promote fair, person-centered, and ethically responsible care [47].

1.8 Dialogue Box: Discussing Ethics, Equity, and Artificial Intelligence in Nursing Practice

(a) Describe how AI is currently used in healthcare and nursing practice.
(b) Identify one real-world example of AI contributing to biased clinical outcomes.
(c) Discuss how structural racism and bias can be embedded in data and algorithm design.

(d) Analyze the role of nurse educators and leaders in identifying and addressing these inequities.
(e) Propose at least two strategies nurse educators can use to prepare nursing students to critically engage with AI in an ethical and equitable manner.
(f) Reflection: In a brief paragraph, reflect on how this assignment has influenced your understanding of nursing's role in shaping equitable healthcare technologies.

1.9 Frameworks for Ethical and Practical AI Integration

While artificial intelligence is increasingly integrated into educational environments, it is unlikely to fully replace human teaching, as the relational, ethical, and critical aspects of education depend on human judgment, empathy, and professional expertise that AI cannot replicate [48]. It is essential that nurse educators approach AI incorporation into curricula, student learning activities, assessments, and evaluations through a structured ethical and practical framework. The rapid evolution of AI technologies, along with concurrent developments in regulatory, legal, and policy environments, has led to the emergence of multiple frameworks designed to guide the responsible adoption of AI in academic settings. This section presents select frameworks that offer foundational strategies for integrating AI into higher education in ways that align with the professional and ethical standards of the nursing discipline.

One significant contribution to this area is the *ETHICAL Principles AI Framework for Higher Education* framework introduced by Wynants and colleagues [49]. The ETHICAL framework stands for Exploration and Evaluation, Transparency and Accountability, Human-Centered Approach, Integrity and Academic Honesty, Continuous Learning and Innovation, Accessibility and Inclusivity, and Legal and Ethical Compliance. This model provides a flexible yet robust foundation that can be tailored to meet the specific needs of diverse educational programs while emphasizing vigilance toward the inherent limitations and biases associated with AI tools. The framework encourages educators to engage in systematic evaluation and critical analysis of AI applications and outputs, to promote transparency and accountability regarding AI use in both educational and administrative contexts, and to prioritize the preservation of human-centered decision-making processes. Furthermore, it underscores the importance of maintaining academic integrity and professionalism when utilizing AI, promoting continuous learning about emerging AI technologies, and ensuring that their implementation advances accessibility and inclusivity. Adherence to applicable legal frameworks and ethical standards remains a central tenet of this approach, reinforcing the need for deliberate and principled AI adoption.

For nurse educators who have already begun to implement AI within their instructional or administrative practices, the *EVERY* Framework, developed by AI for Education and Vera Cubero, offers a reflective structure to ensure continued ethical engagement with AI technologies [50]. The *EVERY* framework represents

Evaluate, Verify, Engage, Revise, and You. This framework advocates a stepwise process whereby users first assess the extent to which AI outputs meet intended pedagogical or operational objectives. It then recommends verification of the accuracy and reliability of information, given the risks of hallucination and embedded bias in AI-generated content. Active engagement with AI tools is encouraged to foster critical oversight and iterative refinement of outputs. Educators are advised to revise AI-assisted work to reflect their academic standards, professional voice, and contextual requirements, recognizing that AI should augment rather than replace human contributions. Finally, the framework stresses personal responsibility for all outputs involving AI, alongside a commitment to transparency regarding the extent and nature of AI's involvement in the educational process.

The framework presented in AI Literacy: A Framework to Understand, Evaluate, and Use Emerging Technology by Angela Elkordy and Ayn Keneman offers a structured approach to developing artificial intelligence (AI) literacy, particularly within educational settings [51]. AI literacy is defined as the capacity to understand, evaluate, and responsibly engage with AI technologies, emphasizing both technical knowledge and critical reflection. This framework is designed to prepare learners and educators to navigate and respond to the increasing influence of AI in various aspects of life and education. Central to the framework are three interconnected domains: understanding AI, evaluating AI, and using AI. The first domain, understanding AI, involves acquiring foundational knowledge of what AI is, how it operates, and how it is embedded in everyday tools and systems. Importantly, it includes recognizing that AI is not neutrality, is shaped by human decisions and may reflect social and cultural biases. The second domain, evaluating AI, emphasizes the development of critical thinking skills to assess the ethical, societal, and individual implications of AI systems. This includes attention to data privacy, algorithmic bias, equity, and the broader consequences of AI implementation. The third domain, using AI, focuses on practical engagement with AI tools, fostering the ability to apply them effectively and ethically in real-world contexts while maintaining human agency and responsibility. Altogether, the framework underscores the importance of AI literacy not merely as a technical skill set, but as a multidimensional competency that integrates ethical reasoning, critical inquiry, and active citizenship. It serves as a guide for educators aiming to equip students with the awareness and skills necessary to interact thoughtfully with AI and to contribute to more just and equitable technological futures.

By adopting similar frameworks, nurse educators are positioned to guide the integration of AI in ways that are thoughtful, principled, and aligned with the ethical foundations of the nursing profession. Such frameworks ensure that AI serves to enhance, rather than undermine, humanistic education and equitable healthcare practice. Examples of frameworks are shown in Table 1.1.

Table 1.1 Ethical and practical AI frameworks in nursing education

Framework	Core components	Primary focus	Application in nursing education
Ethical	Exploration, transparency, human-centeredness, integrity, continuous learning, accessibility, legal compliance	Responsible, ethical AI use in academia	Guides curriculum planning and AI use aligned with nursing ethics
Every	Evaluate, Verify, engage, revise, you	Practical use and personal accountability in AI use	Encourages educators to critically appraise AI content in teaching
AI literacy	Understand AI, evaluate AI, use AI	Building conceptual and critical literacy	Prepares students to analyze, question, and ethically use AI in practice

1.10 Conclusion

This chapter has critically examined how artificial intelligence can be responsibly embedded within nursing education and practice. It highlighted how AI, when guided by ethical principles and informed by nursing values, holds promise for advancing clinical reasoning, promoting health equity, and supporting the professional well-being of nurses. By grounding the discussion in historical developments, educational theory, and moral frameworks, the chapter underscores the need for an intentional and inclusive strategy for AI adoption, one that positions technology as a complementary asset rather than a replacement. Ensuring meaningful integration will require active engagement from nurse educators and leaders to align AI innovations with the realities of nursing practice and the needs of diverse patient populations.

Artificial intelligence is rapidly reshaping the landscape of healthcare and nursing education, offering unprecedented opportunities to enhance clinical reasoning, streamline workflows, and personalized learning. Application of AI in healthcare also presents several significant challenges, such as data privacy concerns, algorithmic bias, health equity issues, cybersecurity risks, and the potential for diagnostic errors [52]. These concerns are similarly reflected in nursing education, where educators must both address these complexities in their curricula and take steps to reduce their influence on student learning and patient care practices. As AI becomes increasingly embedded in educational and clinical settings, nurse educators and healthcare leaders must take proactive roles in guiding its implementation. This includes cultivating digital literacy, fostering ethical awareness, and ensuring that AI tools are designed with input from nurses and aligned with the values of humanistic, patient-centered care. By leveraging ethical frameworks and integrating AI thoughtfully into practice and education, nurses can ensure these tools serve to enhance clinical care and uphold the core values of the profession.

References

1. Alowais SA, Alghamdi SS, Alsuhebany N, Alqahtani T, Alshaya AI, Almohareb SN, et al. Revolutionizing healthcare: the role of artificial intelligence in clinical practice. BMC Med Educ. 2023;23(1):689.
2. Kaul V, Enslin S, Gross SA. History of artificial intelligence in medicine. Gastrointest Endosc. 2020;92(4):807–12.
3. Xu Y, Liu X, Cao X, Huang C, Liu E, Qian S, et al. Artificial intelligence: a powerful paradigm for scientific research. The Innovation. 2021;2(4):100179.
4. Harder N. Advancing healthcare simulation through artificial intelligence and machine learning: exploring innovations. Clin Simul Nurs. 2023;83:101456.
5. Liaw SY, Tan JZ, Lim S, Zhou W, Yap J, Ratan R, et al. Artificial intelligence in virtual reality simulation for interprofessional communication training: mixed method study. Nurse Educ Today. 2023;122:105718.
6. Wangpitipanit S, Lininger J, Anderson N. Exploring the deep learning of artificial intelligence in nursing: a concept analysis with Walker and Avant's approach. BMC Nurs. 2024;23(1):529.
7. Mitha S, Schwartz J, Hobensack M, Cato K, Woo K, Smaldone A, et al. Natural language processing of nursing notes: an integrative review. CIN Comput Inform Nurs. 2023;41(6):377–84.
8. Gao J, Yang Y, Lin P, Park DS. Computer vision in healthcare applications. J Healthc Eng. 2018;2018:5157020.
9. Khalifa M, Albadawy M. AI in diagnostic imaging: Revolutionising accuracy and efficiency. Comput Methods Programs Biomed Update. 2024;5:100146.
10. Wenderott K, Krups J, Zaruchas F, Weigl M. Effects of artificial intelligence implementation on efficiency in medical imaging—a systematic literature review and meta-analysis. NPJ Digit Med. 2024;7(1):265.
11. von Gerich H, Moen H, Block LJ, Chu CH, DeForest H, Hobensack M, et al. Artificial Intelligence-based technologies in nursing: a scoping literature review of the evidence. Int J Nurs Stud. 2022;127:104153.
12. Buchanan C, Howitt ML, Wilson R, Booth RG, Risling T, Bamford M. Predicted influences of artificial intelligence on the domains of nursing: scoping review. JMIR Nurs. 2020;3(1):e23939.
13. Al Khatib I, Ndiaye M. Examining the role of AI in changing the role of nurses in patient care: systematic review. JMIR Nurs. 2025;8(1):e63335.
14. Tighe P, Mossburg S, Gale B. Artificial intelligence and patient safety: promise and challenges. PSNet. 2024;
15. Alderden JG, Johnny JD. Artificial intelligence and the critical care nurse. Vol. 43, Critical Care Nurse. American Association of Critical Care Nurses; 2023.
16. Ronquillo CE, Peltonen LM, Pruinelli L, Chu CH, Bakken S, Beduschi A, et al. Artificial intelligence in nursing: priorities and opportunities from an international invitational think-tank of the nursing and artificial intelligence leadership collaborative. J Adv Nurs. 2021;77(9):3707–17.
17. Dunlap PAB, Michalowski M. Advancing AI data ethics in nursing: future directions for nursing practice, research, and education. JMIR Nurs. 2024;7(1):e62678.
18. Rony MKK, Parvin MR, Ferdousi S. Advancing nursing practice with artificial intelligence: enhancing preparedness for the future. Nurs Open. 2024;11(1):10.1002/nop2.2070.
19. Buchanan C, Howitt ML, Wilson R, Booth RG, Risling T, Bamford M. Predicted influences of artificial intelligence on nursing education: scoping review. JMIR Nurs. 2021;4(1):e23933.
20. Benner P. From novice to expert: excellence and power in clinical nursing practice. Upper Saddle River: Prentice Hall; 2001.
21. Leininger MM, McFarland MR. Madeleine Leininger's theory of culture care diversity and universality. Nurs Theor Nurs Pract. 2010:317–36.
22. Peplau HE. Interpersonal constructs for nursing practice. Nurse Educ Today. 1987;7(5):201–8.
23. Moore EC, Tolley CL, Bates DW, Slight SP. A systematic review of the impact of health information technology on nurses' time. J Am Med Inform Assoc. 2020;27(5):798–807.

24. Bakhoum N, Gerhart C, Schremp E, Jeffrey AD, Anders S, France D, et al. A time and motion analysis of nursing workload and electronic health record use in the emergency department. J Emerg Nurs. 2021;47(5):733–41.
25. Rischel V. Alleviating the burden of documentation to focus on what matters. Inst Healthc Improv. 2022;
26. American Association of Colleges of Nursing (AACN). Domain 10 Personal, Professional, and Leadership Development. [Internet]. American Association of Colleges of Nursing (AACN); 2021 [cited 2025 Apr 6]. Available from: https://www.aacnnursing.org/essentials/tool-kit/domains-concepts/personal-professional-and-leadership-development
27. Rony MKK, Alrazeeni DM, Akter F, Nesa L, Das DC, Uddin MJ, et al. The role of artificial intelligence in enhancing nurses' work-life balance. J Med Surg Public Health. 2024;3:100135.
28. Rodziewicz TL, Houseman B, Hipskind JE. Medical error reduction and prevention. StatPearls Publishing; 2018.
29. Nibbelink CW, Brewer BB. Decision-making in nursing practice: an integrative literature review. J Clin Nurs. 2018;27(5–6):917–28.
30. El Arab RA, Al Moosa OA, Abuadas FH, Somerville J. The role of AI in nursing education and practice: umbrella review. J Med Internet Res. 2025;27:e69881.
31. Chan MMK, Wan AWH, Cheung DSK, Choi EPH, Chan EA, Yorke J, et al. Integration of artificial intelligence in nursing simulation education: a scoping review. Nurse Educ. 2024;50(4):195–200.
32. Rubeis G. The disruptive power of Artificial Intelligence. ethical aspects of gerontechnology in elderly care. Arch Gerontol Geriatr. 2020;91:104186.
33. Randhawa GK, Jackson M. The role of artificial intelligence in learning and professional development for healthcare professionals. Los Angeles: SAGE Publications; 2020. p. 19–24.
34. Papathanasiou IV, Kleisiaris CF, Fradelos EC, Kakou K, Kourkouta L. Critical thinking: the development of an essential skill for nursing students. Acta Inform Medica. 2014;22(4):283.
35. Fakour H, Imani M. Socratic wisdom in the age of AI: a comparative study of ChatGPT and human tutors in enhancing critical thinking skills. In Front Media SA. 2025;10:1528603.
36. Farhud DD, Zokaei S. Ethical issues of artificial intelligence in medicine and healthcare. Iran J Public Health. 2021;50(11):i.
37. Bailey ZD, Krieger N, Agénor M, Graves J, Linos N, Bassett MT. Structural racism and health inequities in the USA: evidence and interventions. The lancet. 2017;389(10077):1453–63.
38. Churchwell K, Elkind MS, Benjamin RM, Carson AP, Chang EK, Lawrence W, et al. Call to action: structural racism as a fundamental driver of health disparities: a presidential advisory from the American Heart Association. Circulation. 2020;142(24):e454–68.
39. Cross JL, Choma MA, Onofrey JA. Bias in medical AI: implications for clinical decision-making. PLOS Digit Health. 2024;3(11):e0000651.
40. Obermeyer Z, Powers B, Mullainathan S. Dissecting racial bias in an algorithm used to manage the health of populations. Science. 2019;366(6464):447–53.
41. Visweswaran S, Sadhu EM, Morris MM, Vis AR, Samayamuthu MJ. Online database of clinical algorithms with race and ethnicity. Sci Rep. 2025;15(1):10913.
42. Vyas D, Eisenstein L, Jones D. Hidden in plain sight–reconsidering the use of race correction in clinical algorithms. N Engl J Med. 2020;383(9):874–82.
43. World Health Organization. Ethics and governance of artificial intelligence for health: large multi-modal models. WHO Guidance; 2024.
44. Stokes F, Palmer A. Artificial intelligence and robotics in nursing: ethics of caring as a guide to dividing tasks between AI and humans. Nurs Philos. 2020;21(4):e12306.
45. OR HB2748: Relating to the use of nursing titles. [Internet]. 2748. 2025. Available from: https://legiscan.com/OR/bill/HB2748/2025
46. Akgun S, Greenhow C. Artificial intelligence in education: addressing ethical challenges in K-12 settings. AI Ethics. 2022;2:431–40.
47. Stokes L. ANA position statement: the ethical use of artificial intelligence in nursing practice. OJIN Online J Issues Nurs [Internet]. 2025;30(2) [cited 2025 Jun 14]. Available from:

https://ojin.nursingworld.org/table-of-contents/volume-30-2025/number-2-may-2025/the-ethical-use-of-artificial-intelligence-in-nursing-practice/

48. Cope B, Kalantzis M, Searsmith D. Artificial Intelligence for education: Knowledge and its assessment in AI-enabled learning ecologies. Educ Philos Theory. 2020;53(12):1229–45.

49. Wynants S, Childers G, De La Torre RY, Budar-Turner D, Vasquez P. ETHICAL principles AI framework for higher education [Internet]. Fullerton: California State University; 2025. [cited 2025 Apr 28]. Available from: https://genai.calstate.edu/communities/faculty/ethical-and-responsible-use-ai/ethical-principles-ai-framework-higher-education

50. AI for Education, Cubero V. How to Use AI Responsibly EVERY Time. AI for Education; 2024.

51. Lee K, Mills K, Ruiz P, Coenraad M, Fusco J, Roschelle J, et al. AI literacy: a framework to understand, evaluate, and use emerging technology; 2024. https://doi.org/10.51388/20.500.12265/218.

52. Bouderhem R. Shaping the future of AI in healthcare through ethics and governance. Humanit Soc Sci Commun. 2024;11(1):1–12.

Olga Kagan and Lilly Mathew

2.1 Introduction

2.1.1 Overview of AI in Nursing Education

Artificial Intelligence (AI) is transforming nursing education by enhancing personalized learning, clinical reasoning, and student engagement. AI-driven tools, including virtual patient simulations, adaptive learning platforms, and intelligent tutoring systems, provide tailored educational experiences, improving knowledge retention and critical thinking skills [1]. These technologies address long-standing challenges in nursing education, such as standardization of curricula and disparities in student readiness. AI-powered virtual simulations allow students to engage with dynamic patient scenarios, offering real-time feedback and individualized learning experiences. These simulations help nursing students develop clinical decision-making skills in a risk-free environment, fostering confidence and preparedness for real-world healthcare settings [2]. Adaptive learning platforms further optimize educational outcomes by analyzing student performance and adjusting content difficulty, ensuring engagement without overwhelming learners. Another critical aspect of AI integration is the use of intelligent tutoring systems, which provide personalized guidance and support based on individual learning styles. These systems mimic human interactions, offering adaptive feedback that enhances knowledge acquisition and competency development.

O. Kagan (✉)
Department of Nursing, Molloy University, Rockville Centre, NY, USA
e-mail: okagan@molloy.edu

L. Mathew
Department of Nursing, Institution: City University of New York School of Professional
Studies, New York, NY, USA
e-mail: lilly.mathew@cuny.edu

D. W. La Rosa et al. (eds.), *Nursing Education in the AI Era*,
https://doi.org/10.1007/978-3-032-12402-9_2

AI-driven approaches also facilitate research and scholarly writing by improving data analysis capabilities, reducing cognitive overload, and supporting literature reviews with advanced retrieval systems [3]. Despite its numerous advantages, AI implementation in nursing education presents challenges, including accessibility disparities, privacy concerns, and the need for faculty training. Faculty members often have concerns about academic integrity with students using AI tools to complete homework and assignments for academic credit. Strategies to overcome these barriers include digital literacy initiatives, infrastructure improvements, and ethical frameworks that ensure responsible AI usage. As AI continues to evolve, its role in nursing education will expand, promoting more efficient, accessible, and equitable learning environments. By integrating AI-driven tools into nursing curricula, educational institutions can bridge gaps in competency development, ensure personalized instruction, and prepare students for the complexities of modern healthcare. AI is not merely a supplement to traditional education, it is reshaping the future of nursing pedagogy and practice, offering scalable solutions for improving educational outcomes and professional readiness.

Nursing education professionals must start thinking about prioritizing investment in artificial intelligence (AI) tools to meet the evolving demands of modern healthcare and enhance the quality of instruction. AI offers transformative benefits such as personalized learning, real-time clinical decision support, and simulation-based training that mirrors complex patient care scenarios. These tools not only improve student engagement and learning outcomes but also prepare future nurses for technology-integrated clinical environments. Moreover, AI can help address faculty shortages and administrative burdens by automating routine tasks, allowing educators to focus on mentorship and critical thinking development. As healthcare systems become increasingly data-driven, integrating AI into nursing curricula ensures that graduates are equipped with the competencies needed for safe, efficient, and equitable care delivery [4]. Recent research studies conducted in this field share valuable insights.

2.1.2 Importance of Integrating AI-Driven Tools for Personalized Learning

Integrating AI-driven tools into nursing education is essential for enhancing personalized learning and improving student outcomes, while keeping in mind ethical considerations, such as privacy and responsible AI implementation, to maximize effectiveness yet maintaining academic integrity [5]. AI facilitates adaptive learning experiences that cater to individual student needs, ensuring optimal engagement and comprehension. Studies emphasize that AI-powered platforms, such as intelligent tutoring systems and gamification-based learning models, enhance student motivation and knowledge retention by dynamically adjusting content difficulty [6].

AI-driven personalization significantly impacts higher education by offering tailored learning experiences based on individual performance metrics. AI's role extends beyond content adaptation—its predictive analytics help identify knowledge gaps, enabling educators to provide targeted interventions and support struggling students effectively. Furthermore, AI fosters innovation in nursing education by promoting critical thinking, problem-solving, and clinical decision-making skills. Its implementation not only improves academic performance but also prepares students for real-world healthcare challenges [7]. As nursing programs continue evolving, leveraging AI-driven learning tools ensures that students receive personalized, efficient, and equitable educational experiences, ultimately strengthening the quality of healthcare education.

2.1.3   Addressing Disparities in Access and Student Readiness

Disparities in access and student readiness for AI-driven technologies in nursing education stem from socioeconomic, technological, and institutional barriers. One of the primary challenges is unequal access to digital infrastructure, particularly in underfunded nursing programs and rural areas, where students face limitations in high-speed internet and AI-based learning tools [1]. Socioeconomic disparities further impact students' ability to afford AI-enhanced resources such as adaptive learning platforms, intelligent tutoring systems, and virtual simulations, resulting in inequitable learning experiences [2]. Additionally, digital literacy gaps remain a pressing issue, with many nursing students and faculty lacking foundational AI knowledge, making it difficult to engage with AI-powered curricula effectively [8]. Institutional readiness also varies, as some nursing programs struggle to integrate AI due to a lack of clear policy frameworks, faculty resistance, and ethical concerns related to student data privacy [3]. Moreover, AI-driven tools may inadvertently reinforce biases, disproportionately affecting students from diverse backgrounds, particularly those with disabilities, who often encounter accessibility barriers (design-related obstacles) in digital learning environments [9]. The unintended consequences of AI adoption, including algorithmic biases and discrepancies in learning accessibility, highlight the importance of equity-focused AI design and ethical oversight [10]. Addressing these disparities requires investment in digital infrastructure, faculty development, and inclusive AI applications to ensure equitable access. Institutions must prioritize AI literacy initiatives, improve accessibility for students with disabilities, and implement ethical frameworks to foster responsible AI use in nursing education. By strategically addressing these challenges, AI can become a transformative force for personalized, equitable learning experiences in nursing education.

2.2   AI-Supported Learning Environment: Competencies and Readiness

2.2.1   Key Skills Required for Educators and Students

The integration of AI into nursing education requires both educators and students to develop essential competencies to maximize its benefits. Educators must possess a strong understanding of AI-driven tools, including adaptive learning platforms, virtual patient simulations, and intelligent tutoring systems, to effectively incorporate them into curricula [3]. Additionally, faculty must be proficient in data interpretation and ethical AI usage to ensure responsible implementation.

To successfully incorporate artificial intelligence (AI) tools into nursing education, faculty must develop a blend of digital fluency, critical thinking, and ethical awareness. This includes understanding how AI functions, evaluating its outputs against clinical evidence, and integrating it meaningfully into curricula to enhance student learning and decision-making skill [4]. Faculty should also be equipped to address ethical concerns such as data privacy, bias, and academic integrity, while fostering a culture of innovation and responsible AI use. Educators should be able to critically assess AI-generated content and teach students to do the same. This involves comparing AI outputs with clinical guidelines and evidence-based practices to ensure safe and accurate decision-making. Programs like the Faculty AI Champion initiative have shown that targeted training can significantly improve educators' confidence and competence in using AI tools for teaching and assessment [11]. Faculty need skills in redesigning curricula to embed AI tools meaningfully. This includes creating assignments that use AI for clinical reasoning, care planning, or patient education, while maintaining academic integrity. Working with IT professionals, data scientists, and healthcare providers can help faculty stay current and effectively implement AI tools in both classroom and clinical settings.

Students, on the other hand, need to develop critical thinking and problem-solving skills to engage with AI-enhanced learning environments effectively. AI literacy, including the ability to evaluate AI-generated recommendations and apply them in clinical scenarios, is crucial for nursing students to enhance their decision-making abilities [2]. Students should also develop competency in data interpretation and digital communication skills, as students will increasingly interact with AI-driven decision support systems and electronic health records. Additionally, students must develop ethical reasoning and professional judgment to navigate issues such as patient privacy, algorithmic bias, and the responsible use of AI in patient care [12]. Finally, adaptability and a growth mindset are vital, enabling students to continuously learn and engage with emerging technologies as they evolve.

2.2.1.1 Digital Literacy and Competency Development

Digital literacy is a fundamental requirement for nursing students and educators to navigate AI-supported learning environments. Competency development should focus on understanding AI algorithms, data security, and ethical considerations in AI-assisted healthcare education [13]. Nursing programs benefit from integrating AI literacy training into curricula to ensure students can critically assess AI-generated insights and apply them effectively in clinical practice. Furthermore, structured AI competency frameworks should be developed to guide educators in implementing AI-driven teaching methodologies while maintaining academic integrity and patient-centered care [3].

In a nursing study that analyzed faculty perceptions found that 82.5% of the faculty were familiar with at least one AI chatbot and acknowledged the benefits of AI chatbots, like enhanced teaching experiences, student engagement, independent learning, and quick access to knowledge. However, they additionally raised concerns about misinformation, reduced faculty-student interaction, inadequacies in addressing complex clinical scenarios, legal and ethical issues, and misuse of information [14].

2.2.2 Strategies for Overcoming Barriers to AI Adoption

Overcoming barriers to AI adoption in nursing education requires targeted strategies to ensure equitable access, faculty readiness, and ethical implementation. Institutions must invest in digital infrastructure, providing reliable internet access, AI-compatible devices, and well-equipped computer labs, particularly in underfunded nursing programs [15, 16]. Financial support programs, such as grants and subsidies, can help students afford AI-driven learning tools, reducing socioeconomic disparities. Faculty training initiatives are essential to fostering AI literacy, ensuring educators can integrate AI seamlessly into curricula. Structured workshops and continuing education programs can equip faculty with the skills needed to navigate AI-powered platforms and enhance student engagement [17]. Embedding digital literacy training into nursing education further supports student readiness, enabling them to interpret AI-generated data and apply AI-assisted clinical decision-making tools effectively. Addressing ethical concerns surrounding AI bias and data privacy is critical for responsible AI implementation. Institutions should establish clear guidelines to mitigate algorithmic bias and ensure secure handling of student data [18]. Transparency in AI applications, along with continuous monitoring, can enhance trust and promote equitable learning experiences. By prioritizing infrastructure development, faculty training, digital literacy initiatives, and ethical AI policies, nursing programs can bridge accessibility gaps and foster a more inclusive and technologically proficient educational environment.

2.3   AI-Driven Tools in Nursing Programs

2.3.1   Virtual Patient Simulations

AI-driven virtual patient simulations have revolutionized nursing education by enhancing clinical reasoning, boosting student confidence, and improving preparedness for real-world scenarios. These simulations create realistic patient encounters, allowing students to engage in dynamic decision-making processes. By continuously adjusting complexity based on student responses, virtual simulations help refine diagnostic skills and critical thinking [19].

Virtual reality (VR)-based simulations enable nursing students to interact with lifelike scenarios that mimic real clinical settings. This exposure reduces anxiety and increases self-assurance, particularly in high-stress medical situations [20]. Studies indicate that immersive VR simulations contribute to higher engagement levels and better knowledge retention compared to traditional methods [21]. Additionally, AI-driven simulators provide individualized feedback, allowing students to identify errors and improve performance in a controlled environment [22]. These technologies also play a critical role in preparing students for emergency and critical care situations. The ability to repeatedly engage in simulated high-risk scenarios enhances competency in clinical decision-making, leading to improved patient outcomes in real-life practice [23]. Furthermore, AI-powered gamification elements in simulations promote an interactive and personalized learning experience, encouraging student motivation and skill development [5]. As nursing programs continue to incorporate AI-driven virtual simulations, the benefits extend beyond technical proficiency—students gain confidence, adaptability, and preparedness for evolving healthcare environments. Ensuring accessibility and proper faculty training in AI-enhanced learning remains crucial for maximizing its impact in nursing education.

2.3.2   Adaptive Learning Platforms

AI-driven adaptive learning platforms are transforming nursing education by personalizing instruction based on student progress, ensuring tailored learning experiences that enhance knowledge retention and skill acquisition. These platforms use artificial intelligence to analyze student performance, identify strengths and weaknesses, and adjust educational content accordingly [24]. Through continuous feedback and customized learning pathways, students receive appropriate challenges without experiencing cognitive overload, ultimately improving engagement and academic outcomes [19].

Case studies illustrate the effectiveness of adaptive learning in nursing education. Andersen et al. [25] conducted a scoping review demonstrating how blended adaptive learning technologies improved clinical reasoning and decision-making skills. Nursing students using AI-powered platforms showed increased confidence in managing complex patient cases, particularly in simulation-based assessments. Similarly, Gao performed a meta-analysis on adaptive learning systems, highlighting their role in enhancing student performance across various healthcare disciplines [26]. The study found that nursing students experienced improved exam scores and clinical competency through AI-driven individualized learning approaches. By integrating adaptive learning technology, nursing education can ensure that students progress at a pace aligned with their learning needs while strengthening essential competencies. Institutional investments in AI-driven platforms and faculty training are necessary to maximize these benefits and support continuous learning in nursing curricula.

2.3.3   Intelligent Tutoring Systems

AI-driven Intelligent Tutoring Systems (ITS) are transforming nursing education by providing personalized feedback, tailored learning experiences, and fostering the development of clinical decision-making skills. These systems use machine learning algorithms to adapt educational content based on individual student progress, ensuring that learners receive customized instruction suited to their needs [27]. By analyzing student responses in real-time, ITS platforms can identify knowledge gaps and provide targeted remediation, improving competency in critical nursing concepts. The ability of ITS to support clinical reasoning is particularly valuable in nursing education, where decision-making is fundamental to patient care. Studies have shown that AI-powered tutoring systems enhance problem-solving abilities by simulating real-world healthcare scenarios and guiding students through evidence-based approaches [7]. For example, research on ITS implementation in nursing programs demonstrated improved diagnostic accuracy and faster response times among students engaging with adaptive learning modules. Additionally, ITS fosters independent learning and skill refinement, empowering students to take ownership of their educational journey. By offering immediate feedback and personalized guidance, ITS minimizes reliance on instructor-led interventions and enhances student confidence [28]. This approach has been shown to increase engagement and knowledge retention, particularly in complex clinical subjects. Furthermore, ITS systems contribute to educational equity by providing consistent learning opportunities regardless of geographic or socioeconomic barriers [29]. As nursing programs continue to integrate AI-driven ITS, their potential to refine clinical judgment and enhance educational outcomes will grow. Investing in faculty training and digital literacy initiatives is essential to ensuring ITS technologies are effectively incorporated into curricula, optimizing their impact on nursing education.

2.4   Personalizing Education with AI

2.4.1   Using AI to Refine Instructional Strategies

AI-driven personalized education in nursing enhances instructional strategies, improves student engagement and knowledge retention, and addresses disparities in learning opportunities. Adaptive learning platforms refine instructional approaches by tailoring content based on individual progress, ensuring students receive appropriately challenging material without cognitive overload [24]. AI-powered simulations allow students to practice clinical decision-making in realistic scenarios, reinforcing critical thinking and problem-solving skills [30].

2.4.2   Improving Knowledge Retention and Student Engagement

AI also improves student engagement by utilizing gamification elements, interactive assessments, and immersive virtual environments that cater to diverse learning styles [19]. Personalized AI-driven feedback supports knowledge retention by pinpointing learning gaps and providing targeted support [27]. Studies show that AI-integrated learning environments foster higher motivation and participation, leading to improved academic performance [25].

> In a nursing study, Chat-GPT intervention group that received an "Artificial Intelligence Integrated Nursing Process" training showed improvement in problem-solving skills, an increase in positive attitudes towards AI, and a significant increase in their nursing process competency and satisfaction levels than the control group [31].

2.4.3   Addressing Disparities Through Targeted Interventions

To address disparities, AI tools offer multilingual support and accessibility features that enable inclusive learning for students from varied backgrounds [32]. AI analytics identify students at risk, allowing educators to implement interventions that ensure equitable support and prevent learning disadvantages [17]. Additionally, AI-powered remote learning expands access to quality nursing education for students in underserved regions, improving overall educational equity [33]. By integrating AI into nursing education, institutions can enhance personalized learning experiences, promote student success, and bridge educational gaps effectively.

2.5   AI Integration into Nursing Curricula

2.5.1   Examples of AI Tools Used in Current Nursing Programs

Integrating AI-driven tools such as virtual patient simulations, adaptive learning platforms, and intelligent tutoring systems (ITS) into nursing curricula requires a strategic and phased approach. The key to successful implementation lies in seamlessly aligning these technologies with existing learning objectives and teaching methodologies (Table 2.1). Measuring the effectiveness of integrated AI tools should include both quantitative and qualitative methods. Conduct observations, and interviews as well as analyze metrics such as completion rates, accuracy scores, and time spent on tasks to gain insights into individual student progress. Compare learning outcomes achieved using AI-driven tools with those obtained through traditional teaching methods to determine the platform's relative effectiveness.

Table 2.1 Teaching methods

Teaching method	Brief description (citation)	Examples
Thayer method	An instructor-guided approach originating from West Point Academy (1820). It requires rigorous pre-class preparation and uses in-class problem-solving and discussion to deepen understanding [34, 35]	Student "brief the bot" explaining what prompt they used to generate AI output to their question and why the answer is correct or not. This creates AI use transparency, helps with AI literacy, and critical thinking
Flipped classroom	A method where students review instructional content (e.g., video lectures, readings) on their own before class and then engage in interactive, application-based activities during class time [36, 37]	Students develop content-based learning module or seminar aligned with the learning objectives for a class on a selected topic using approved AI platforms ethically, including but not limited to video avatars, animations, video or image generation tools.
Active learning	An umbrella term for strategies that incorporate activities such as group work, discussions, and hands-on exercises to shift the focus from passive lectures to student engagement and deeper comprehension [38]	Active learning involves engaging with AI tools in developing creative deliverables using institutionally approved generative AI chatbots such as Microsoft Co-pilot or Google Gemini
Problem-based learning (PBL)	A student-centered method in which learners collaborate to solve real-world, complex problems. This process enhances critical thinking, problem-solving skills, and self-directed learning by placing students in charge [39, 40]	Each student to consult with approved AI tools to generate ideas or develop programs or solutions to problems experienced by vulnerable populations

(continued)

Table 2.1 (continued)

Teaching method	Brief description (citation)	Examples
Team-based learning (TBL)	A structured small-group instructional strategy that involves individual preparation followed by team activities to solve problems, ensuring accountability and fostering collaborative learning [41]	A group of students to consult with approved AI tools to generate ideas or develop programs or solutions to problems experienced by vulnerable populations, or communities
Socratic method	A dialectical approach based on asking guided, probing questions that challenge assumptions and stimulate critical thinking and reflective dialogue [42]	Probing prompts with a chatbot to stimulate critical thinking on a topic where students can converse with AI using peer-reviewed literature to guide the dialogue
Inquiry-based learning	An approach that emphasizes investigation and exploration. Students pose questions, conduct research, and engage in collaborative problem solving to construct their own understanding of a subject [43]	Explore AI prompts to construct and develop a body of knowledge on a particular topic of interest using AI-enabled research tools like Claude, Covidence, Researchrabbit.ai, SCISPACE, and others approved AI tools
Experiential learning	A process where learners gain knowledge through direct experience, reflection, and application of theory in real-world or simulated settings. This "learning by doing" is central to personal and professional growth [44, 45]	Employ AI-driven scenarios for nursing simulation using virtual reality (VR), mixed reality (MR), augmented reality (AR) and other

2.5.2 Faculty Development and Institutional Support

Successful AI integration requires ongoing faculty development programs to enhance educators' competency in AI-driven pedagogy. To achieve this, institutions must provide training workshops on using AI tools for assessment and instruction, ensuring faculty can effectively implement technology-based learning strategies [7] and ethical guidelines for AI adoption, addressing concerns about data security and bias.

To successfully incorporate AI into nursing curricula, institutions should begin with pilot programs to evaluate effectiveness and scalability [5]. Faculty must receive continuous training and support in AI adoption, ensuring seamless integration into coursework. Developing interdisciplinary AI literacy courses within nursing curricula can enhance student familiarity with AI applications in healthcare [46]. Additionally, expanding access to AI-enhanced learning tools, such as virtual reality interventions, ensures students gain hands-on experience with advanced clinical technologies [47].

Faculty can refine their use of virtual simulations and ITS by aligning content with specific learning outcomes, reinforcing competency-based education [48]. Further, collaboration between nursing programs and AI developers can refine educational technologies, ensuring they align with competency-based learning goals [49].

In a recently completed Faculty AI champion project, the findings indicated increased faculty understanding of AI and improved self-efficacy in identifying, locating, and evaluating AI tools. Participants reported a rise in their AI knowledge (mean score: pre 3.4 to post 4.25/5) and gave the program a strong endorsement (avg. rating: 9.5/10) [50]. Field notes highlighted enthusiasm for AI integration in health professions education, with faculty aiming to expand their knowledge and explore practical applications for teaching. The program serves as a model for ethical and effective AI integration in nursing education.

2.6   AI-Supported Research and Scholarly Writing

2.6.1   Leveraging AI for Literature Reviews and Data Analysis

Artificial intelligence has revolutionized academic research by streamlining literature reviews and enhancing data analysis in nursing studies. AI-powered tools assist researchers in quickly identifying relevant literature, extracting key findings, and synthesizing information, significantly reducing manual effort and improving the efficiency of systematic reviews [51]. Machine learning algorithms facilitate the analysis of large datasets, enabling nursing researchers to identify trends and correlations that inform evidence-based practice [52]. Additionally, generative AI tools support scholarly writing by assisting in the development of research summaries and organizing references effectively [53]. There are several journals, professional organizations, websites, and conferences where news about AI-driven tools is discussed and disseminated (Table 2.2).

2.6.2   Ethical Considerations in AI-Assisted Research

While AI offers numerous advantages in scholarly writing, its integration into research raises important ethical concerns. The risk of AI-generated misinformation, biases in algorithmic recommendations, and potential issues with academic integrity must be addressed [54]. Researchers must ensure transparency in AI-generated outputs, validating data sources and cross-referencing results to maintain accuracy. Ethical guidelines for AI-assisted writing should emphasize responsible citation practices and prevent over-reliance on AI-generated content without human verification [55]. Furthermore, maintaining authorship integrity in AI-assisted academic work is crucial, ensuring researchers maintain critical engagement with their findings rather than accepting AI-generated insights without scrutiny [49].

Table 2.2 Resources

Category	Resource	Description
Websites and online resources	National Library of Medicine (NLM)	Database of biomedical literature, including articles on AI in nursing education. Offers advanced search filters
	PubMed Central (PMC)	Free-access repository of biomedical and life sciences journal literature, including AI applications in healthcare
	IEEE Xplore Digital Library	Archives technical research on AI in healthcare and education, emphasizing AI algorithms and their implementation
	Professional Nursing Organizations	Sites like the American Nurses Association (ANA) provide articles, reports, and ethical perspectives on AI in nursing
Journals and publications	Journal of Nursing Education	Publishes research on AI-driven teaching methodologies and advancements in nursing education
	Computers, Informatics, Nursing (CIN)	Covers technological applications, including AI, in nursing practice and education
	Applied Artificial Intelligence	Features research on AI algorithms and their practical applications in healthcare education
	Journal of Nursing Informatics JMIR Publications	Offers nursing continuing professional development activities, regular columns, and articles impacting nurse informaticists Digital health journal offering peer-reviewed articles on AI's role in healthcare and medical education
Books and monographs	AI in Healthcare, AI in Education	Books provide in-depth insights into AI integration. Search springer, Elsevier, Wiley for reputable sources
	Natural Language Processing & Machine Learning	Books on AI techniques relevant to nursing education, like chatbots and personalized learning models
Professional organizations and conferences	American Nurses Association (ANA)	Offers publications and updates on AI technology in nursing practice and education
	Association for the Advancement of Artificial Intelligence (AAAI)	Provides AI research and development updates, including educational applications
	International Conferences on AI in Education (AIED)	Gathers global researchers to discuss AI advancements in education
	Health Information Management Systems Society (HIMSS)	Healthcare IT organization covering AI applications in healthcare technology
Government agencies and funding	National Institutes of Health (NIH)	Supports AI research projects in healthcare; provides funding opportunities for advancements in medical AI applications

2.6.3 Future Directions for AI-Driven Academic Work

The future of AI-driven scholarly writing in nursing education will likely focus on refining AI models to enhance their accuracy and reliability in research applications. Advanced AI tools are expected to play a greater role in personalized research assistance, tailoring literature reviews and recommendations based on individual research interests [56]. As AI technologies evolve, interdisciplinary collaborations between nursing researchers and AI developers will be essential in ensuring AI tools align with evidence-based practice and ethical standards [57]. Additionally, AI-assisted peer review processes may emerge to streamline the publication of nursing research while maintaining rigorous academic scrutiny [1].

2.7 Conclusion

The integration of artificial intelligence (AI) into nursing education offers transformative potential, enhancing the quality and effectiveness of teaching and learning. AI tools such as intelligent tutoring systems, personalized learning platforms, and virtual reality simulations provide individualized learning pathways, adaptive assessments, and immediate feedback, catering to diverse learning styles and ensuring optimal knowledge retention. Moreover, AI chatbot tools can enhance student scholarly work by offering assistance with writing and giving insights into their work, and can assist in editing and sharpening their writing skills. However, successful implementation requires careful planning, robust infrastructure, comprehensive training programs, and ongoing evaluation. Addressing challenges such as faculty resistance, data privacy and security, and equitable access to technology is crucial for maximizing the benefits of AI in nursing education. Ethical considerations, including mitigating algorithmic bias and ensuring transparency, are paramount to fostering trust and confidence in AI-powered systems. By strategically leveraging AI's strengths and addressing its limitations, nursing programs can enhance their assessment processes, improve student learning outcomes, and prepare the next generation of nurses for the rapidly evolving healthcare landscape. The journey towards integrating AI into nursing education is ongoing, requiring continuous adaptation, collaboration, and a commitment to excellence.

Note the teaching method and related examples in Table 2.1 and the resources located in Table 2.2.

References

1. El Arab R, Al Moosa O, Abuadas F, Somerville J. The role of AI in nursing education and practice: umbrella review. J Med Internet Res. 2025;27:e69881. https://www.jmir.org/2025/1/e69881. https://doi.org/10.2196/69881.
2. Abualrahi A, Habobi S, Almutar S, Al-Khwaildi F, Alalq M, Bomurah R, Abdrabalnabi Z, Al-habib E, Al-Mahdi F, Al-Sadah F. Paradigm shift: a systematic review of integrating artificial intelligence in nursing education. Am J Nurs Res. 2024;12(3):50–6. https://pubs.sciepub.com/ajnr/12/3/2/index.html

3. Shen M, Shen Y, Liu F, Jin J. Prompts, privacy, and personalized learning: integrating AI into nursing education—a qualitative study. BMC Nurs. 2025;24(1):470. https://bmcnurs.biomed-central.com/articles/10.1186/s12912-025-03115-8

4. O'Connor S, Peltonen L-M, Topaz M, Chen L-YA, Michalowski M, Ronquillo C, Stiglic G, Chu CH, Hui V, Denis-Lalonde D. Prompt engineering when using generative AI in nursing education. Nurse Educ Pract. 2024;74:103825. https://doi.org/10.1016/j.nepr.2023.103825.

5. Nguyen KV. The use of generative AI tools in higher education: ethical and pedagogical principles. J Acad Ethics [Internet]. 2025 [Cited 2025 May 6]; Available from: https://doi.org/10.1007/s10805-025-09607-1.

6. Abbes F, Bennani S, Maalel A. Generative AI and gamification for personalized learning: literature review and future challenges. SN Comput Sci. 2024;5(8):1154. https://link.springer.com/article/10.1007/s42979-024-03491-z

7. Treve M. Integrating artificial intelligence in education: impacts on student learning and innovation. Int J Vocat Educ Train Res. 2024;10(2):61–9. https://www.researchgate.net/publication/387776580_Integrating_Artificial_Intelligence_in_Education_Impacts_on_Student_Learning_and_Innovation

8. Shao KZ, Wilson D, Cho EKM, Tang S, Ma H, Makhsous S. Bridging educational equity gaps: a systematic review of AI-driven and new technologies for students living with disabilities in STEM education. In 2025. [cited 2025 May 6]. Available from: https://peer.asee.org/bridging-educational-equity-gaps-a-systematic-review-of-ai-driven-and-new-technologies-for-students-living-with-disabilities-in-stem-education

9. Simms RC. Generative artificial intelligence (AI) literacy in nursing education: a crucial call to action. Nurse Educ Today. 2025;146:106544. https://pubmed.ncbi.nlm.nih.gov/39708405/

10. Stanford.edu. Is AI exacerbating disparities in education? [Internet]. Available from: https://news.stanford.edu/stories/2024/09/educating-ai

11. Ronquillo C, Topaz M, Peltonen L-M, O'Connor S, Borycki E. Artificial intelligence and nursing: priorities and opportunities in education. J Nurs Scholarsh. 2023;55(2):125–33. https://doi.org/10.1111/jnu.12838.

12. Nashwan AJ, Abujaber AA. Embracing artificial intelligence in nursing education: preparing future nurses for a technologically advanced healthcare landscape. Evid Based Nurs. 2024;28(1):23–4. https://doi.org/10.1136/ebnurs-2023-103906.

13. Atkins RL, Brown KM, Mudd SS, Ghobadi K, Baker DJ, Szanton S. Transforming nursing education: AI and competency-based learning for an inclusive and equitable future [Internet]. Rochester: Social Science Research Network; 2024. [cited 2025 May 6]. Available from: https://papers.ssrn.com/abstract=4988538

14. Saleh ZT, Rababa M, Elshatarat RA, Alharbi M, Alhumaidi BN, Al-Za'areer MS, et al. Exploring faculty perceptions and concerns regarding artificial intelligence Chatbots in nursing education: potential benefits and limitations. BMC Nurs. 2025;24(1):440. Available from https://bmcnurs.biomedcentral.com/articles/10.1186/s12912-025-03082-0

15. Marr B. Forbes. [cited 2025 May 6]. 11 Barriers to effective AI adoption and how to overcome them. Available from: https://www.forbes.com/sites/bernardmarr/2024/05/10/11-barriers-to-effective-ai-adoption-and-how-to-overcome-them/

16. Alotaibi N, Wilson CB, Traynor M. Enhancing digital readiness and capability in healthcare: a systematic review of interventions, barriers, and facilitators. BMC Health Serv Res. 2025;25(1):500. Available from https://bmchealthservres.biomedcentral.com/articles/10.1186/s12913-025-12663-3

17. Bubb AJ. Forbes. [cited 2025 May 6]. Unlocking AI's potential: overcoming barriers to adoption. Available from: https://www.forbes.com/councils/forbestechcouncil/2025/02/21/unlocking-ais-potential-overcoming-barriers-to-adoption/

18. Edmondson J. Breaking down barriers to AI adoption: overcoming challenges in implementing artificial intelligence [Internet]. Businesstechweeklycom 2022 [cited 2025 May 6]. Available from: https://www.businesstechweekly.com/operational-efficiency/artificial-intelligence/barriers-to-ai-adoption/

19. Murugan T, Periasamy K, Abirami AM. Adopting artificial intelligence tools in higher education: student assessment. Boca Raton: CRC Press; 2025.
20. Kirthika KM, Sangeetha S, Immanual R, Sanjana N. Current state of AR and VR in healthcare. In: Augmented wellness: exploring the power of VR and AR in healthcare. Springer; 2025. https://link.springer.com/chapter/10.1007/978-981-96-2952-7_10.
21. Bandari P, Alkrida AA, Athiraja A, Alharbi AA, Rajeswaran N. Exploring virtual reality's impact on medical education in healthcare: a comprehensive overview. In: Augmented wellness. Springer; 2025. https://link.springer.com/chapter/10.1007/978-981-96-2952-7_8.
22. Gunturu V, Krishnamoorthy R, Tanaka K, Alla PCR, Ramesh JVN, Ravichandran S. Energy efficient: analysis of virtual reality (VR) and augmented reality (AR) in modern healthcare systems. In: Augmented wellness. Springer; 2025. https://link.springer.com/chapter/10.1007/978-981-96-2952-7_5.
23. Saxena A, Thukral P. Science behind augmented reality and virtual reality in healthcare. In: Augmented wellness. Springer; 2025. https://link.springer.com/chapter/10.1007/978-981-96-2952-7_6.
24. Gligorea I, Cioca M, Oancea R, Gorski AT, Gorski H, Tudorache P. Using artificial intelligence in e-learning: a literature review. Educ Sci. 2023;13(12):1216. https://www.mdpi.com/2227-7102/13/12/1216
25. Andersen BL, Jørnø RL, Nortvig AM. Blending adaptive learning technology into nursing education: a scoping review. Contemp Educ Technol. 2021;14(1):ep333. https://www.cedtech.net/download/blending-adaptive-learning-technology-into-nursing-education-a-scoping-review-11370.pdf
26. Gao Y. The potential of adaptive learning systems to enhance learning outcomes: a meta-analysis. https://era.library.ualberta.ca/items/e8de2f25-be42-4c7b-967a-510fa4bf98a8
27. Faisal SM, Khan W, Ishrat M. AI-driven pedagogy and assessment in TVET: transforming education through AI – enhancing pedagogy and assessment in TVET. IGI Global Scientific Publishing; 2025. https://www.igi-global.com/chapter/ai-driven-pedagogy-and-assessment-in-tvet/377115
28. Alkhuwaylidee AR, Gatea AK, Alomari MF. Smarter learning environment: exploring the need for an intelligent tutoring system in Iraqi universities. In: Current and future trends on AI applications: volume 1. Springer; 2025. https://link.springer.com/chapter/10.1007/978-3-031-75091-5_5.
29. Merino-Campos C. The impact of artificial intelligence on personalized learning in higher education: a systematic review. Trends High Educ. 2025;4(2):17. https://doi.org/10.3390/higheredu4020017.
30. Jyothi V, Chintamaneni V, Sravani D, Jaffar AY, Alwabli A, Rajeswaran N. Virtual reality-based intelligent internet of medical things health monitoring system: in future aspects. In: Augmented wellness. Springer; 2025.
31. Arkan B, Dallı ÖE, Varol B. The impact of ChatGPT training in the nursing process on nursing students' problem-solving skills, attitudes towards artificial intelligence, competency, and satisfaction levels: single-blind randomized controlled study. Nurse Educ Today. 2025;152:106765. https://www.sciencedirect.com/science/article/abs/pii/S0260691725002011?via%3Dihub
32. Kumar R, Kumar P, Sobin CC, Subheesh NP, editors. Blockchain and AI in shaping the modern education system. Boca Raton: CRC Press; 2025.
33. Owan VJ, Abang KB, Idika DO, Etta EO, Bassey BA. Exploring the potential of artificial intelligence tools in educational measurement and assessment. Eurasia J Math Sci Tech Ed. 2023;19(8):em2307. https://www.ejmste.com/article/exploring-the-potential-of-artificial-intelligence-tools-in-educational-measurement-and-assessment-13428
34. Shell GR. Teaching and learning through case method. Boston: Harvard Business School Publishing; 2002.
35. Van Dam K, Schipper M, Buskens E. The Thayer Method: a historical and pedagogical analysis. J Educ Methods. 2019;45(3):215–29.

36. Erbil DG. A review of flipped classroom studies: is there consistent evidence about the benefits? Educ Technol Res Dev. 2020;68(2):333–56.
37. Lo CK, Hew KF. Flipped classroom pedagogy: a meta-analysis. J Educ Comput Res. 2017;55(1):1–26.
38. Freeman S, Eddy SL, McDonough M, Smith MK, Okoroafor N, Jordt H, et al. Active learning increases student performance in science, engineering, and mathematics. Proc Natl Acad Sci USA. 2014;111(23):8410–5.
39. Savery JR. Overview of problem-based learning: definitions and distinctions. Interdiscip J Probl-Based Learn. 2006;1(1):9–20.
40. Barrows HS, Tamblyn RM. Problem-based learning: an approach to medical education. New York: Springer; 1980.
41. Parmelee DX, Michaelsen LK, Cook S, Hudes P. Team-based learning: a practical guide for implementation in medical education. Med Teach. 2012;34(5):275–8.
42. Jones K. The Socratic method in legal education: implementing reflective dialogue. Law Teach. 2006;40(1):72–87.
43. Justice C, Rice J, Warry W, Inglis S, Miller S, Sammon S. Inquiry-based learning: a conceptual framework. High Educ. 2007;54(5):693–705.
44. Hendrix EA. Experiential learning: best practices for student engagement and knowledge retention. J Exp Educ. 2014;82(1):25–36.
45. Kolb DA. Experiential learning: experience as the source of learning and development. Englewood Cliffs: Prentice Hall; 1984.
46. Zhai X, Zhao R, Jiang Y, Wu H. Unpacking the dynamics of AI-based language learning: flow, grit, and resilience in Chinese EFL contexts. Behav Sci (Basel). 2024;14(9):838. https://www.mdpi.com/2076-328X/14/9/838
47. Padmapriya S, Torne P, Ray AP, Gupta A, Anand R, Jain V. Virtual reality mental health interventions: AR/VR solutions for well-being. In: Augmented wellness. Springer; 2025. https://link.springer.com/chapter/10.1007/978-981-96-2952-7_1.
48. Rezaeikhonakdar D, Wrigley J, Shaw RJ. Policy recommendations to facilitate nurse-driven optimization of clinical artificial intelligence tools. CIN: Comput Inform Nurs. 2024;42(5):320. https://journals.lww.com/cinjournal/citation/2024/05000/policy_recommendations_to_facilitate_nurse_driven.2.aspx
49. Ghimire A, Qiu Y. Redefining pedagogy with artificial intelligence: how nursing students are shaping the future of learning. Nurse Educ Pract. 2025;84:104330. https://archive.hshsl.umaryland.edu/server/api/core/bitstreams/0594b167-3800-40ce-bae5-cd33e0625c66/content
50. Bunnell DJ, Fisher CA, Stephens C, Quattrini V, Roesch A. Productivity and pedagogy: faculty AI champions program outcomes. Baltimore, School of Nursing: Poster presented at the University of Maryland; 2024.
51. Bolaños F, Salatino A, Osborne F, Motta E. Artificial intelligence for literature reviews: opportunities and challenges. Artif Intell Rev. 2024;57(10):259. https://link.springer.com/article/10.1007/s10462-024-10902-3
52. Kitsios F, Kamariotou M, Syngelakis AI, Talias MA. Recent advances of artificial intelligence in healthcare: a systematic literature review. Appl Sci. 2023;13(13):7479. https://www.mdpi.com/2076-3417/13/13/7479
53. Mozelius P, Humble N. On the use of generative AI for literature reviews: an exploration of tools and techniques. In: European conference on research methodology for business and management studies; 2024. https://papers.academic-conferences.org/index.php/ecrm/article/view/2528.
54. Cheng A, Calhoun A, Reedy G. Artificial intelligence-assisted academic writing: recommendations for ethical use. Adv Simul. 2025;10(1):22. https://advancesinsimulation.biomedcentral.com/articles/10.1186/s41077-025-00350-6
55. Kuteeva M, Andersson M. Diversity and standards in writing for publication in the age of AI—between a rock and a hard place. Appl Linguist. 2024;45(3):561–7. https://doi.org/10.1093/applin/amae025.

56. Kovalainen T, Pramila-Savukoski S, Kuivila HM, Juntunen J, Jarva E, Rasi M, et al. Utilising artificial intelligence in developing education of health sciences higher education: an umbrella review of reviews. Nurse Educ Today. 2025;147:106600. Available from https://www.science-direct.com/science/article/pii/S0260691725000358?via%3Dihub

57. Whig P, Sharma P, Aneja N, Elngar AA, Silva N, editors. Artificial intelligence and machine learning for sustainable development: innovations, challenges, and applications. Boca Raton: CRC Press; 2024. doi:https://doi.org/10.1201/9781003497189

Ethical Considerations in AI Integration

3

Renee McLeod-Sordjan

3.1 Introduction: Ethical AI in Nursing Education

Artificial intelligence (AI) is rapidly transforming healthcare delivery, clinical decision-making, and health education. From predictive analytics, diagnostic interpretation, virtual simulation, to personalized learning, AI technologies are becoming embedded in the educational infrastructure of nursing programs. As these tools evolve, they offer unprecedented opportunities to enhance learner engagement, tailor instruction, and improve workforce readiness. However, the integration of AI into nursing education raises complex ethical concerns that must be addressed to ensure that technological innovation aligns with core ethical values of the nursing profession, such as justice, autonomy, integrity, and respect for human dignity.

At the heart of these concerns is the potential for AI systems to perpetuate existing inequities. Algorithmic bias, often embedded in the data used to train AI models, can lead to disparities in both educational and healthcare outcomes. Additionally, the increasing reliance on data intensive technologies heightens the risk of privacy violations and opaque decision-making processes. These risks are particularly troubling in nursing education, where fairness, inclusivity, and trust are foundational to professional formation and safe practice. Evidence-based nursing practice is reliant on analysis of best evidence and scientific inquiry.

This chapter critically examines the ethical landscape of AI in nursing education. It is organized around four interrelated themes: (a) addressing algorithmic bias, data privacy, transparency, and cautionary principles; (b) mitigating AI's potential to reinforce bias; (c) ensuring equity and fairness in AI-enhanced educational settings; and (d) navigating the emerging landscape of policy guidance and regulatory frameworks. Together, these themes underscore the urgent need for nurse educators and

R. McLeod-Sordjan (✉)
Department of Nursing, Morehouse School of Medicine, Atlanta, GA, USA
e-mail: rmcleodsordjan@msm.edu

D. W. La Rosa et al. (eds.), *Nursing Education in the AI Era*,
https://doi.org/10.1007/978-3-032-12402-9_3

35

academic leaders to engage thoughtfully with AI's ethical implications and develop strategies that promote just and equitable learning environments. Current workforce efficiency requires nurses to be prepared for the enhanced technological processes required for complex health care. Not aligning curricula with advancements will exacerbate the knowledge-to-practice gap.

3.2   Attitudes Related to AI Use

Integrating artificial intelligence (AI) into health professions education, particularly nursing, has generated a range of attitudes among educators, students, and institutions, reflecting optimism and ethical caution. Generally, attitudes toward AI in nursing education are cautiously optimistic, with widespread acknowledgment of its transformative potential alongside persistent ethical, technical, and pedagogical concerns. Attitudes toward AI in nursing and health professions education reflect a nuanced balance of enthusiasm and skepticism, grounded in both empirical findings and conceptual analysis. Studies employing surveys, interviews, and systematic reviews reveal patterns in how educators, students, and institutions perceive AI integration into curricula and practice.

Wang et al. [1] conducted a cross-sectional survey across four academic institutions in China to assess the knowledge, attitudes, and concerns of 1243 participants, including nursing students, clinical faculty, and AI professionals, regarding the integration of artificial intelligence (AI) into nursing practice. Over 70% of respondents agreed that AI has the potential to enhance clinical decision-making and improve educational outcomes. However, 46% expressed concern about the lack of clear regulatory frameworks and the ethical implications of AI, particularly with respect to data privacy, algorithmic bias, and broader issues in medical ethics. Respondents emphasized uncertainty around accountability in AI-assisted care, transparency in machine-led decisions, and the potential erosion of humanistic elements in nursing. Using a validated questionnaire with Likert-scale items, the study applied multivariable regression models to identify predictors of positive attitudes. Key facilitators included prior exposure to AI tools and strong institutional support for digital innovation.

A parallel study in the United States by Olson et al. [2] explored similar themes within a different cultural and educational context, focusing specifically on nurse anesthesia students and faculty. Their findings revealed both alignment and divergence from Wang et al.'s results. While a majority of U.S. participants acknowledged AI's potential to streamline perioperative decision-making and optimize anesthesia delivery, concerns remained regarding AI's capacity to fully account for the nuance and complexity of clinical judgment in high-stakes environments. Like their Chinese counterparts, participants in the Olson et al. study expressed ethical reservations, particularly around issues of accountability, potential deskilling, and the devaluation of patient-centered care. Interestingly, the study noted generational and role-based differences, with students more likely to express enthusiasm for AI integration, while faculty were more cautious, citing the need for clearer educational frameworks, ethical guidelines, and interdisciplinary dialogue. These parallel findings underscore the global relevance of AI in nursing education while highlighting the importance of localized strategies that consider professional roles, training context, and regulatory environments.

Similarly, Couper [3] reinforces these findings, emphasizing that AI integration in nursing education holds transformative potential through personalized learning, AI-enhanced simulation, and real-time performance analytics. However, it also presents critical ethical and infrastructural challenges. Privacy risks related to student data collection, the danger of embedded bias in AI algorithms, and the threat of exacerbating educational inequities due to disparities in access to technology permeate attitudes of both students and faculty. Alruwaili et al. [4], in a descriptive cross-sectional design of 220 nurses in Saudi Arabia, supported this perception as novice nurses had more conservative attitudes toward AI than undergraduate nursing students, with significant differences observed based on gender ($\chi^2 = 4.67$, $p < 0.05$). Couper [3] highlights the necessity for ethical governance, including transparency, accountability, and alignment with established privacy laws, as foundational to ethically integrating AI in nursing education. Resistance among faculty and students rooted in fear of role displacement and insufficient digital fluency further underscores the need for robust training and clear communication about AI's role as a complement to, rather than a replacement for, human educators.

Castonguay et al. [5] echo the ambivalence surrounding AI, particularly in the context of generative technologies like ChatGPT. Their reflection underscores that while students are increasingly curious about the innovative possibilities of AI in content generation and real-time feedback, faculty remain wary of academic integrity violations, erosion of critical thinking, and the challenge of developing updated pedagogical frameworks. De Gagne, Hwang, and Jung [6] add a cyber ethics lens, illustrating that attitudes are influenced by broader concerns over surveillance, autonomy, and equity, especially when AI tools become embedded in evaluation systems. Collectively, these findings illustrate that while stakeholders acknowledge the potential of AI to support nursing education and clinical judgment, the technology must be approached with humility, regulation, and a deep commitment to human-centered values.

To contextualize these findings globally, several systematic reviews and research findings demonstrate that ethical attitudes are evolving, raising additional desires for strategic institutional readiness that include policy frameworks and faculty development. Badawy, Zinhom, and Shaban [8], in a systematic review of 43 studies across multiple countries, found that *over 60% of the literature emphasized ethical ambiguity* surrounding AI's role in clinical judgment, particularly when algorithms conflict with professional nursing values. This uncertainty fostered calls for *clear institutional guidelines and interdisciplinary ethics training* to mitigate moral distress among nurses. The review also highlighted that only *18% of the institutions reviewed had established ethical frameworks or protocols for AI deployment*, suggesting a significant policy gap despite growing awareness.

Similarly, Buchanan et al. [9] in a scoping review of 87 publications, predicted that AI will increasingly influence all five core domains of nursing (*clinical practice, education, administration, research, and policy*) yet found that nurses frequently report discomfort due to *lack of training and unclear ethical boundaries*, particularly in areas like automated triage and predictive analytics. While both reviews acknowledge AI's potential to enhance care efficiency and safety, they converge on the conclusion that *attitudinal hesitancy is strongly correlated with institutional unpreparedness.* The studies emphasize the need for strategic readiness through faculty development, updated curricula, and ethical guidance, aligning closely with the patterns observed in survey data such as Wang et al. [1] and concerns raised by Couper [3].

To further develop the discussion on evolving ethical attitudes and institutional readiness regarding AI in nursing education, several studies and reviews offer nuanced perspectives. Gonzalez-Garcia et al. [10] conducted a cross-sectional study exploring the impact of ChatGPT usage on nursing students. The findings revealed that 73.2% of respondents had used ChatGPT, and among them, 85.7% found it beneficial for academic performance. However, ethical concerns remained: 67.4% of students were worried about academic integrity, and 51.5% expressed uncertainty about the accuracy and transparency of ChatGPT-generated content. These concerns indicate a simultaneous appreciation of AI's utility and a desire for clear usage guidelines and training to ensure ethical integration into academic practice. Complementing this, Saleh et al. [11] examined faculty perceptions of AI Chatbots in nursing education. Faculty recognized benefits like enhanced engagement and immediate feedback, but expressed significant concerns related to data privacy, dependency on AI tools, and potential loss of critical thinking skills among students. Notably, over 70% emphasized the need for institutional frameworks to guide AI use, pointing to a broader call for structured policies and support mechanisms.

In summary, these studies demonstrate that attitudes toward AI in nursing and health professions education are shaped by multiple factors, including user experience, institutional context, ethical concerns, and the perceived alignment of AI tools with pedagogical goals. Future efforts to foster acceptance and effective use of AI must focus on faculty training, inclusive policy development, and empirically grounded strategies that safeguard humanistic values in health professions education. Moreover, there is a shared acknowledgment of AI's potential in educational innovation, coupled with ethical apprehensions that demand institutional foresight. Faculty and student perceptions converge on the necessity for transparent policies, digital literacy training, and a reaffirmation of humanistic values in nursing education. Current literature strengthens the argument for proactive curriculum development and ethical governance as foundational components of AI integration.

3.3   Potential for Impacting Nursing Student Learner Outcomes

Integrating artificial intelligence (AI) into nursing education offers transformative potential for learner outcomes, as it introduces novel tools for knowledge acquisition, clinical reasoning, and ethical discernment. Bozic [12] emphasizes that AI technologies, when meaningfully incorporated into educational settings, can significantly improve engagement, efficiency, and the personalization of instruction. For example, adaptive learning platforms powered by AI can offer tailored content based on individual student progress, while virtual simulations with AI-driven patient avatars allow students to practice and refine clinical skills in realistic, low-risk environments. Bozic [12] also highlights how AI can foster evidence-based thinking by facilitating access to large data sets and decision-support systems. These innovations, he argues, support deeper learning and better preparation for technology-rich clinical environments, aligning nursing education with the demands of twenty-first-century healthcare.

Bozic [12] proposes a structured framework for integrating AI into the nursing curriculum, emphasizing a progressive and ethically grounded approach. His model advocates for a three-tiered curriculum that begins with foundational AI literacy, ensuring students grasp core concepts such as machine learning, data inputs, and algorithmic function. The second tier focuses on applied knowledge through simulated clinical decision-making and AI-enhanced diagnostic reasoning. This phase aims to build student confidence in using AI tools as supportive mechanisms in patient care rather than replacements for clinical judgment. The final tier introduces critical discussions on ethical, legal, and professional implications, including data privacy, bias mitigation, and the nurse's accountability when interfacing with AI systems. Bozic [12] underscores the importance of aligning AI education with nursing values, positioning AI not as a disruption but as a complementary force in preparing future-ready nurses.

The broader literature reinforces Bozic's model and demonstrates how AI's implementation in nursing education can shape outcomes across cognitive, psychomotor, and affective domains. Yasin et al. [13] through a scoping review, found that AI-assisted tools improved nursing students' performance in clinical judgment and diagnostic accuracy. Their analysis of AI integration across global nursing programs revealed that students using AI-supported learning platforms showed stronger retention of clinical content and higher confidence in patient care simulations. Moreover, the review emphasized the importance of institutional capacity-building, particularly in faculty readiness and infrastructure, to sustain long-term educational benefits.

In their umbrella review, El Arab et al. [14] further documented the pedagogical impact of AI in nursing and healthcare education, citing significant gains in learner motivation, self-regulated learning, and real-time formative assessment. Their synthesis of over 30 studies highlighted AI's ability to support individualized learning plans and reduce faculty workload without compromising instructional quality. The authors stress, however, that the benefits of AI must be balanced with robust ethical training and oversight mechanisms. Without such a balance, disparities in access and digital fluency could exacerbate educational inequalities.

Complementing these findings, Farooqi et al. [15], Khreisat et al. [16], and Yelne et al. [17] each emphasize that AI integration must be accompanied by thoughtful attention to governance, transparency, and bias mitigation. Their systematic reviews reveal widespread concern about unregulated use of AI in instructional settings and advocate for cross-sector policy frameworks that establish standards for data ethics, privacy, and inclusivity. This body of work reinforces the view that while AI is a powerful tool for enhancing learner outcomes, its success hinges on institutional alignment, faculty preparedness, and ethical stewardship.

3.4 Ethical Concerns of AI

Ethical issues surrounding artificial intelligence (AI) in nursing education are multifaceted and increasingly documented in both empirical research and conceptual analyses. Central concerns include algorithmic bias, data privacy, lack of transparency, and the erosion of humanistic care principles. De Gagne et al. [18] emphasize the need for "cyberethics" in nursing education, warning that without intentional ethical frameworks, AI could reproduce social and cultural biases embedded in training data, disproportionately disadvantaging marginalized groups. Similarly, Watson [19] identifies risks in AI-driven informatics systems that automate learning assessments without sufficient human oversight, potentially compromising fairness and student autonomy. The World Health Organization [20] and the American Nurses Association [21] have both issued guidance advocating for the integration of ethical governance, transparency, and accountability mechanisms in AI systems used in healthcare and education. Chaudhry, Cukurova, and Luckin [22] also propose a transparency index for AI in education, arguing that open communication about AI decision-making processes is essential to ethical deployment. Collectively, ethical frameworks suggest robust faculty training, clear institutional policies, and student empowerment to ensure AI enhances rather than undermines nursing education's ethical and humanistic foundations see Table 3.1.

The Ethical AI in Nursing Education Domains and Strategies Framework (see Table 3.1) offers a structured approach to guiding the responsible integration of artificial intelligence into academic environments. It organizes ethical priorities into three core domains: *Transparency, Fairness and Inclusion,* and *Data Privacy.*

Table 3.1 Ethical AI in nursing education—domains and strategies framework

Domain	Key focus areas	Representative strategies
Transparency	Explainable AI Open communication Clear decision-making	Integrate AI models that allow users to understand outcomes Promote dialogue around AI use Ensure clarity in AI-supported decisions
Fairness and inclusion	Mitigating algorithmic bias Inclusive curriculum Equitable resource access	Audit and address biases in datasets Embed diversity in case examples and design Provide fair access to AI tools and learning environments
Data privacy	Secure and confidential use Informed consent Data protection policies	Use encrypted platforms for data sharing Obtain consent for data usage in education Implement and enforce data governance policies

Within the domain of transparency, the framework encourages the adoption of explainable AI systems, open communication, and clear decision-making processes, ensuring that students and educators understand how AI tools generate outcomes and influence learning. The fairness and inclusion domain addresses the mitigation of algorithmic bias, calls for integrating diverse perspectives in curricular content, and promotes equitable access to AI-enhanced educational resources. In the realm of data privacy, the framework underscores the importance of secure platforms, informed consent for data use, and robust institutional data protection policies. Together, these strategies serve as actionable ethical guardrails, aligning technological advancement with the values of nursing education and protecting both learners and patients.

The integration of artificial intelligence (AI) into nursing education and clinical practice presents unprecedented opportunities for innovation and efficiency, yet it also raises complex ethical concerns that must be critically addressed. As AI systems become more embedded in healthcare decision-making and educational assessment, concerns around fairness, autonomy, and accountability have intensified. Scholars and practitioners alike emphasize that without rigorous ethical oversight, AI tools risk reinforcing existing disparities, compromising patient and learner privacy, and undermining the humanistic values foundational to nursing. These concerns are not merely theoretical; they are substantiated by emerging evidence that reveals concrete risks tied to algorithmic bias, inadequate data protections, and opaque decision-making processes. Ethical integration of AI requires intentional efforts to identify these risks and to implement frameworks that uphold professional integrity, social justice, and the rights of both learners and patients.

3.4.1 Algorithmic Bias

- *Focus:* Identify, assess, and mitigate biases in AI systems.

Algorithmic bias presents a serious challenge to equity and fairness in nursing education. AI systems, particularly those relying on historical or poorly curated datasets, risk perpetuating existing disparities. Bias can enter at multiple points in AI processes:

- *Data collection*, where training sets may overrepresent certain populations (e.g., White, English-speaking patients) and underrepresent others (e.g., rural or non-English-speaking communities).
- *Design*, where developers' assumptions or lack of interdisciplinary input may embed unexamined values or reinforce dominant cultural norms and.
- *Deployment*, where AI tools are used in contexts that differ from those they were developed for, potentially magnifying disparities.

For example, an AI grading system designed using data from students at highly resourced universities might assess participation or written communication in ways that penalize students from underrepresented backgrounds or non-native English speakers. Farooqi et al. [15] found that AI tools used in academic assessments may unintentionally favor students from well-resourced backgrounds, reflecting underlying data imbalances. Yelne et al. [17] echoed these concerns, pointing to disparities in AI-assisted learning modules that reinforce linguistic and cultural biases. From a clinical training perspective, if an AI tool used to support diagnostic reasoning has been trained on electronic health records predominantly from urban, insured populations, its predictive accuracy may drop when applied in rural or underserved settings, potentially misleading students or faculty in decision-making exercises.

To bring this to life for learners, educators might:

- *Case Example 1:* Present students with two patient scenarios processed by an AI triage tool; one from an urban, insured White male and one from a rural, uninsured Latina woman. Learners can be asked to analyze discrepancies in the AI's risk assessments and discuss possible sources of bias in the algorithm.
- *Case Example 2:* Faculty can be shown an AI-based essay scoring tool that rates submissions differently based on sentence structure or word choice, and lead a discussion on how cultural communication styles can influence outcomes and what equitable grading practices might look like.

De Gagne [18] emphasized the importance of regular audits and validation testing to ensure algorithmic outputs are evidence-based and equitable. Embedding bias recognition modules into nursing curricula and faculty training can prepare educators to critically assess the tools they use and adapt pedagogical strategies accordingly. By equipping nurse educators with the language and tools to interrogate bias, nursing education can support more inclusive, just, and data-conscious AI implementation.

3.4.2 Data Privacy

- *Focus:* Ensure confidentiality and security of personal and sensitive data.

The collection and analysis of student data through AI systems raise critical ethical and legal issues. Khreisat et al. [15] identified unauthorized surveillance, continuous tracking, and the commodification of student data as serious privacy threats. Dankwa-Mullan [23] argued for policy mechanisms that mirror HIPAA-like protections in educational settings, while the World Health Organization [20] urged governments to implement global standards for AI data governance. These protections are vital when AI tools are used for formative and summative evaluations, as breaches can compromise student trust, well-being, and academic integrity. Strategies to mitigate privacy risks include anonymizing data, encrypting communications, and offering opt-out options for AI-assisted interventions.

In education, AI poses threats to transparency and explainability when utilized for regulatory decisions. One of the central ethical challenges is the "black box" phenomenon, in which the internal logic of an AI system (e.g., how it scores a student's performance or flags academic dishonesty) is not easily interpretable, even by its developers. This opacity can undermine trust and due process, particularly when AI is used in high-stakes decisions like grading, admissions, or disciplinary actions. Such systems can obscure the rationale behind educational outcomes, leaving students and faculty unable to contest or understand how decisions are made [24]. Students cannot challenge algorithmic biases and errors without explainability. This becomes especially problematic in light of the Family Educational Rights and Privacy Act (FERPA), which guarantees students the right to inspect and request correction of their educational records. Zelde [25] argues that AI tools used in online proctoring and behavioral monitoring may collect and analyze biometric, keystroke, or webcam data without students' full understanding or consent, raising serious concerns about privacy, bias, and the lack of clear procedural protections.

However, AI also holds the potential to *enhance* compliance and fairness when implemented ethically. For instance, well-designed AI systems can automate documentation for accreditation or support early alerts for at-risk students, allowing institutions to intervene equitably and in line with regulatory mandates. When algorithms are transparent, regularly audited, and subject to human oversight, they can promote consistent enforcement of institutional policies and reduce ad hoc or biased decision-making. To meet ethical and legal obligations, especially under FERPA, institutions must ensure AI tools are interpretable, their data use is clearly disclosed, and students are informed of their rights. Promoting algorithmic transparency and procedural fairness is essential to aligning AI adoption with both ethical imperatives and educational law.

3.4.3 Transparency

- *Focus:* Open communication about AI decision-making processes.

Transparency is essential for building trust in AI-enhanced nursing education. Chaudhry et al. [22] developed a Transparency Index Framework that helps assess how openly AI systems communicate their decision-making logic. Without transparency, students and faculty may become overly reliant on tools they do not fully understand, leading to cognitive passivity. Riess [26] advocated for explainable AI (XAI) models that provide detailed rationales for automated feedback or assessment outcomes. De Gagne et al. [27] recommended integrating reflective activities into AI curricula, allowing students to question the reliability and implications of machine-generated guidance. Transparency not only aids understanding but also promotes accountability in AI use.

3.5   Practical Implementation (Connected to Each Ethical Concern)

3.5.1   Mitigating Bias

Educators can play a pivotal role in mitigating algorithmic bias through structured training and curriculum design. Yasin et al. [13] proposed incorporating ethical impact assessments as part of the institutional review process for adopting new technologies. These assessments evaluate whether the AI tools align with pedagogical objectives and uphold standards of justice. Additionally, the American Nurses Association [21] recommends professional development courses focusing on detecting and responding to AI-related biases. Hoelscher et al. [28] utilized the mnemonic NURSES to summarize the ANA position statement on ethical use of AI. Competencies include basic knowledge of AI concepts; data interpretation, analysis, and evaluating data quality; ethical implications of AI; critical judgment of AI-generated recommendations; and collaborative communication. By equipping faculty with these competencies, institutions foster environments where technology supports, rather than undermines, diversity, and inclusion.

- *Mitigating Bias Strategies:*
  - Rubrics for recognizing and reducing inherent bias.
  - Training modules for nurse educators on ethical AI use.
  - Institutional support for faculty workload related to training/committees.

3.5.2   Ensuring Equity and Fairness

To ensure equitable access to AI-enhanced learning, nursing programs must adopt inclusive design principles. El Arab et al. [14] advocate for multilingual learning tools, culturally relevant content, and flexible assessment methods that reflect students' varied experiences. Eden et al. [29] presented case studies from low-resource settings demonstrating how low-bandwidth, mobile-friendly AI platforms could expand access to simulation-based learning. Programs must also ensure that AI does not inadvertently penalize students with limited digital literacy. Equity can be embedded through universal design for learning (UDL), peer support models, and institutional policies that prevent discrimination based on technology access.

- *Ensuring Equity and Fairness Strategies:*
  - Developing inclusive curricula that promote fairness in AI-enhanced education.
  - Case studies and real-world examples.

3.5.3 Enhancing Transparency

AI transparency can be advanced through both technical and pedagogical strategies. Bozic [12] proposed incorporating annotated AI simulations that display reasoning steps, confidence levels, and data sources. Ibuki et al. [30] suggested offering students opportunities to reverse-engineer AI outputs during lab sessions to foster deeper understanding. Incorporating reverse-engineering of AI outputs into lab sessions offers a dynamic way to build students' critical thinking, AI literacy, and ethical awareness. In this approach, students interact with AI tools, such as diagnostic systems, grading algorithms, or language models, not merely as users but as analysts. By observing how AI systems respond to different inputs and experimenting with modifications (e.g., changing a patient's age or altering the tone of an essay), students begin to uncover the hidden logic behind AI decisions. This hands-on process allows them to hypothesize which variables the algorithm is prioritizing and validate those hypotheses through additional test cases, effectively treating the model as a "black box" they are tasked with decoding.

These exercises also open a valuable space for ethical reflection. Instructors can prompt students to consider whether the AI exhibited bias, whether its decisions would hold up under legal scrutiny (such as FERPA's amendment rights), and how a lack of transparency might impact fairness or accountability. Discussions grounded in a reverse-engineering experience make abstract concerns like algorithmic bias or explainability more concrete and actionable. As a result, students not only gain technical insights but also develop a deeper understanding of how AI can both support and challenge educational and clinical integrity. Johnson et al. [7] emphasized that such practices also benefit clinical decision-making by ensuring nurses can validate or contest AI recommendations. Transparency thus becomes a learning objective in itself, one that cultivates critical thinking and ethical reflection.

- *Enhancing Transparency Strategies:*
  - Creation of tools and practices for demystifying AI processes in education.
  - Engage students in reverse engineering exercises, simulations, and assignments.

3.6   Policy and Regulatory Guidance

As artificial intelligence (AI) becomes more embedded in nursing education, the need for coherent policies, regulatory safeguards, and faculty support mechanisms grows increasingly urgent. The rapid pace of innovation risks has outpaced ethical and institutional readiness, especially in academic environments traditionally centered around human-centric pedagogy. Robust policy guidance is essential not only to protect students and patients but also to ensure equitable implementation, reduce disparities, and build confidence among educators. Regulatory frameworks and professional standards must evolve in tandem with technological capabilities to ensure that AI tools uphold nursing's ethical values, legal responsibilities, and academic integrity. This section outlines three key policy-related areas: ethical frameworks, regulatory guidelines, and educator support systems.

Ethical Frameworks and Best Practices

Ethical frameworks provide foundational guidance for responsible AI adoption in nursing education. The World Health Organization [20] advocates for embedding ethical principles such as autonomy, beneficence, non-maleficence, and justice directly into educational and institutional AI strategies. These principles serve as a moral compass, especially when AI is used in high-stakes decision-making scenarios like risk prediction, student evaluation, or simulation training. Konidena et al. [31] propose a dual-level model of implementation, suggesting that institutions address ethics both at the macro level through policy and governance, and at the micro level through curriculum design. They recommend using case-based instruction and problem-based learning to engage students in ethical reflection on real-world dilemmas, such as whether AI should override a nurse's clinical judgment in alert systems. Eden et al. [29] reinforce this approach by calling for an integration of ethics modules across all levels of nursing education to help learners internalize critical ethical reasoning in the age of intelligent technologies.

Regulatory Guidelines and Policy Guidance

National and institutional policy guidance plays a vital role in creating accountability and standards of safety. The American Nurses Association [21] offers a position statement outlining conditions under which AI may be ethically and safely used in clinical and academic settings. Their recommendations include maintaining human oversight over automated decisions, ensuring transparency of algorithmic logic, and implementing clear opt-out procedures for students and patients alike. Watson [19] further argues that accrediting bodies should embed AI ethics into institutional review criteria, requiring programs to demonstrate both technical competence and ethical preparedness. Chaudhry et al. [22] call for transparency mechanisms such as third-party algorithm audits and public reporting on AI outcomes to prevent algorithmic harm. These efforts reflect a broader shift toward governance structures that can adapt to the dynamic nature of AI technologies, while reinforcing public trust and professional accountability.

Educator Support

Across recent scholarship, the integration of artificial intelligence (AI) in nursing education and practice is portrayed as both promising and fraught with complex ethical, pedagogical, and infrastructural challenges. Al-Hassan et al. [32] suggest that AI can enable pedagogical innovations like adaptive tutoring, but also warn that a lack of faculty preparedness and institutional support hinders meaningful integration. Sustained educator development is the linchpin for ethical and effective AI integration. As noted by Molyneux [33]· faculty are often underprepared to interpret, apply, or critique AI tools within pedagogical frameworks. Without proper support, well-intentioned innovations may falter or introduce unintended ethical risks.

Wei et al. [34] expand on these concerns by noting that the success of AI in clinical education depends heavily on its contextual alignment with nursing workflows, faculty training, and interdisciplinary collaboration. Chu et al. [35] advocate for tiered faculty development initiatives, ranging from foundational workshops on AI principles to advanced certification programs in AI and data ethics. Peer mentoring and interdisciplinary learning communities also offer valuable models for ongoing support. These structures allow early adopters to guide their peers through technological onboarding, ethical scenario planning, and curriculum design. Additionally, institutional investment is needed to allocate protected time, technical infrastructure, and continuing education resources so that educators can remain agile in a rapidly evolving digital landscape. Faculty training should not be viewed as a one-time intervention but as a continuous, iterative process aligned with the nursing profession's ethical and social responsibilities.

3.7 Illustrative Use Cases to Integrate AI Ethically

While robust policy frameworks and faculty development initiatives form the structural foundation for ethical AI integration, their real-world value is realized through application in diverse educational settings. To bridge the gap between policy and practice, it is critical to illustrate how educators, policymakers, and AI developers can operationalize these principles in day-to-day academic and professional contexts. The following use cases provide concrete examples of how the ethical, regulatory, and pedagogical guidance outlined above can be translated into meaningful action: shaping curricula, informing institutional strategy, and guiding the development of responsible AI tools that align with the values of nursing education. *See* Table 3.2 *for suggested key focus areas and teaching practices.*

Ethical Teaching Practices for AI in Nursing Education (see Table 3.2) outlines practical strategies for embedding ethical principles into the design and delivery of nursing curricula. It highlights three key pillars: *Curriculum Integration, Policy and Regulatory Guidance,* and *Continuous Professional Development. These pillars are* each essential to fostering ethical AI literacy among educators and students. Curriculum integration involves the use of case studies, role-playing, and critical discussions to help learners engage with real-world dilemmas involving AI, such as bias in clinical decision tools or privacy concerns in AI-based simulations. Policy

Table 3.2 Ethical teaching practices for AI in nursing education

Curriculum integration	Policy and regulatory guidance	Continuous professional development
Case studies in ethical AI	Institutional guidelines	Workshops and seminars on AI ethics
Role-playing and simulations	National and international policies	Ongoing training and educational resources
Critical discussions and ethical debates	Ethical frameworks and best practices	Collaborative learning communities

and regulatory guidance ensure that teaching practices are grounded in institutional, national, and international standards, helping faculty navigate the complex legal and ethical terrain of AI technologies. Finally, continuous professional development supports faculty through structured workshops, seminars, and collaborative learning communities, enabling them to remain current on ethical trends and best practices. This triad approach ensures that ethical AI education is not a one-time initiative, but an evolving, system-wide commitment embedded at every level of nursing instruction.

The following are use cases to illustrate Table II for educators, nurses, and policy makers.

For Educators Use The Ethical AI in Nursing Education Domains and Strategies Framework to guide curriculum development that integrates ethical considerations into nursing education.

3.7.1 Use Case 1: For Educators Integrating Ethical AI into Nursing Curricula

Audience Undergraduate and Graduate Nursing Faculty.

Goal Embed ethical AI principles into teaching practice using simulation, case-based learning, and critical dialogue.

Application
A graduate nursing professor designs a simulation-based course module where students interact with AI-enabled clinical decision support tools. As part of the curriculum, students engage in structured role-play exercises where they must decide whether to override or follow AI-generated treatment recommendations. These simulations are accompanied by critical discussions exploring the ethical implications of algorithmic bias, data transparency, and professional accountability.

For undergraduates, instructors incorporate guided case studies on AI triage systems or wearable health devices, using them to introduce principles like informed consent and data privacy. These exercises are mapped to AACN Essentials and QSEN competencies, ensuring alignment with core professional outcomes.

Impact Students demonstrate greater ethical reasoning in tech-enabled clinical scenarios, preparing them for AI-integrated healthcare settings.

For Policy Makers Reference the framework to align AI regulations with ethical educational practices.

3.8   Use Case 2: For Policy Makers Aligning Nursing Education Policy with AI Ethics

Audience Academic Deans, Accreditation Bodies, Nursing Boards, Legislators

Goal Ensure regulatory alignment with ethical and educational standards for AI use.

Application
A state board of nursing revises its program accreditation standards to include guidelines on ethical AI integration. Drawing from the WHO's[20] ethical principles (2024), ANA's policy recommendations [21], and the institution's framework, the board, school, or curriculum committee mandates that all accredited programs show evidence of curriculum elements addressing algorithmic bias, data protection, and AI transparency.Similarly, a nursing school faculty develops institutional policy to require all new course proposals involving technology to pass through an AI ethics review committee. This ensures curriculum-level compliance with national and international ethical norms and promotes standardized language and expectations across programs.

Impact Ethical AI becomes a codified expectation in nursing education, reducing legal risk and enhancing public trust.

For AI Clinical Nurses Apply the ANA [21] policy recommendations and The Ethical AI in Nursing Education Domains and Strategies Framework to evaluate and adjust AI applications ensuring ethical compliance.

3.8.1   Use Case 3: For AI Clinical Nurse Designing Nursing-Compatible Ethical AI Tools

Audience AI Developers, EdTech Vendors, Informatics Specialists, Nurses.

Goal Ensure that AI tools used in nursing education meet ethical and pedagogical requirements.

Application
An AI developer collaborates with nurse informaticists and bedside nurses on an adaptive testing platform for nursing programs and consults the Ethical AI in Nursing Education Domains and Strategies Framework to design algorithm transparency features. These include explainable feedback loops that allow faculty and students to understand how the system evaluates clinical reasoning.

During beta testing, the company partners with a graduate nursing program to pilot the tool and collects feedback via faculty workshops and student focus groups, ensuring alignment with ethical teaching practices. Developers use this input to improve fairness and reduce cultural or linguistic bias in scoring rubrics.

Impact Nursing educators gain access to ethically robust AI technologies that enhance learning without compromising professional standards.

3.9 Conclusion

In conclusion, the integration of artificial intelligence into nursing education is not as radical a departure as it may seem. Technology has long been a part of academic evolution, from the early adoption of simulation technology, writing aids (e.g., word processors), to the widespread use of computers. AI represents the next phase in this continuum, offering sophisticated tools that can personalize learning, enhance clinical reasoning, and support data-informed decision-making. However, with these advancements come complex ethical challenges that require careful navigation. As AI reshapes pedagogical practices and clinical preparation, nursing educators, institutions, and policymakers must respond with intentional strategies that prioritize transparency, fairness, and accountability. By adopting ethical frameworks, enacting regulatory safeguards, and investing in educator development, the nursing profession can harness AI's potential to enrich learning while upholding its core values of compassion, justice, and patient-centered care. Future efforts must remain interdisciplinary and inclusive, ensuring that AI enhances, not replaces, the human dimensions of nursing education. This ethical vigilance is essential to preparing a nursing workforce equipped to lead in an increasingly digital healthcare landscape.

References

1. Wang X, Fei F, Wei J, Huang M, Xiang F, Tu J, Wang Y, Gan J. Knowledge and attitudes toward artificial intelligence in nursing among various categories of professionals in China: a cross-sectional study. Front Public Health. 2024;12:1433252.
2. Olson J, Thiel L, Ko A, Mason J, Olla P. Nurse anesthesia student and faculty attitudes on artificial intelligence. J Nurs Anesth Educ. 2025; https://doi.org/10.63524/jnae.129203.
3. Couper AL. Challenges and opportunities of artificial intelligence in nursing education. J Nurs Rep Clin Pract. 2025;3(2):213–5.
4. Alruwaili MM, Abuadas FH, Alsadi M, Alruwaili AN, Ramadan OEM, Shaban M, et al. Exploring nurses' awareness and attitudes toward artificial intelligence: implications for nursing practice. Digit Health. 2024;10:20552076241271803. https://doi.org/10.1177/20552076241271803.
5. Castonguay A, Farthing P, Davies S, Vogelsang L. Revolutionizing nursing education through AI integration: a reflection on the disruptive impact of ChatGPT. Nurse Educ Pract. 2023;72:103450.
6. De Gagne J C, Hwang H, Jung D. Cyberethics in nursing education: ethical implications of artificial intelligence. Nurs Ethics. 2024 Jun;31(6):1021–30. https://doi.org/10.1177/09697330231201901.

7. Johnson EA, Dudding KM, Carrington JM. When to err is inhuman: an examination of the influence of artificial intelligence-driven nursing care on patient safety. Nurs Inq. 2024 Jan;31(1):e12583.

8. Badawy W, Zinhom H, Shaban M. Navigating ethical considerations in the use of artificial intelligence for patient care: a systematic review. Int Nurs Rev. 2024;72(3):e13059.

9. Buchanan C, Howitt ML, Wilson R, Booth RG, Risling T, Bamford M. Predicted influences of artificial intelligence on the domains of nursing: scoping review. JMIR Nurs. 2020;3(1):e23939. https://doi.org/10.2196/23939.

10. Gonzalez-Garcia A, Bermejo-Martinez D, Lopez-Alonso AI, Trevisson-Redondo B, Martín-Vázquez C, Perez-Gonzalez S. Impact of ChatGPT usage on nursing students education: a cross-sectional study. Heliyon. 2025;11(1):e41559.

11. Saleh ZT, Rababa M, Elshatarat RA, Alharbi M, Alhumaidi BN, Al-Za'areer MS, Jarrad RA, Al Niarat TF, Almagharbeh WT, Al-Sayaghi KM, Fadila DE. Exploring faculty perceptions and concerns regarding artificial intelligence Chatbots in nursing education: potential benefits and limitations. BMC Nurs. 2025;24(1):440.

12. Božić V. Artificial intelligence in nurse education. Eng Appl Artif Intell. 2024;132:107629.

13. Yasin YM, Al-Hamad A, Metersky K, Kehyayan V. Incorporation of artificial intelligence into nursing research: a scoping review. Int Nurs Rev. 2024;72(1):e13084. https://doi.org/10.1111/inr.13013.

14. El Arab RA, Al Moosa OA, Abuadas FH, Somerville J. The role of AI in nursing education and practice: umbrella review. J Med Internet Res. 2025;27:e69881.

15. Farooqi MTK, Amanat I, Awan SM. Ethical considerations and challenges in the integration of artificial intelligence in education: a systematic review. J Excellence Manag Sci. 2024;3(4):35–50. https://doi.org/10.69565/jems.v3i4.314.

16. Khreisat MN, Khilani D, Rusho MA, Karkkulainen EA, Tabuena AC, Uberas AD. Ethical implications of AI integration in educational decision making: systematic review. Educ Admin Theor Pract. 2024;30(5):8521–7. https://doi.org/10.53555/kuey.v30i5.4406.

17. Yelne S, Chaudhary M, Dod K, Sayyad A, Sharma R. Harnessing the power of AI: a comprehensive review of its impact and challenges in nursing science and healthcare. Cureus. 2023;15(11):e49252. https://doi.org/10.7759/cureus.49252.

18. De Gagne JC. The state of artificial intelligence in nursing education: past, present, and future directions. Int J Environ Res Public Health. 2023;20(6):4884.

19. Watson AL. Ethical considerations for artificial intelligence use in nursing informatics. Nurs Ethics. 2024 Sep;31(6):1031–40. https://doi.org/10.1177/09697330241230515.

20. World Health Organization. Ethics & governance of WHO-endorsed AI for healthcare: guidance for governments and institutions. Geneva: WHO; 2024.

21. American Nurses Association Center for Ethics and Human Rights. The ethical use of artificial intelligence in nursing practice [Internet]. Silver Spring (MD): ANA; 2022. [cited 2025 May 10]. Available from: The Ethical Use of Artificial Intelligence in Nursing Practice. https://www.nursingworld.org/~48f653/globalassets/practiceandpolicy/nursing-excellence/ana-position-statements/the-ethical-use-ofartificial-intelligence-in-nursing-practice_bod-approved-12_20_22.pdf.

22. Chaudhry MA, Cukurova M, Luckin R. A transparency index framework for AI in education. In: International conference on artificial intelligence in education. Cham: Springer; 2022. p. 195–8.

23. Dankwa-Mullan I. Health equity and ethical considerations in using artificial intelligence in public health and medicine. Prev Chronic Dis. 2024;21:E64.

24. Chauhan S, Dutta A. Artificial intelligence in student privacy and data security. Int J Adv Res Comput Sci. 2025;16(3):146–51.

25. Zeide E. Big proctor: online proctoring problems and how FERPA can promote student data due process. Notre Dame J on Emerging Technol. 2022;3:74.

26. Riess DL. Integrating artificial intelligence ethically in nursing education. Nursing. 2025;55(4):56–60.

27. De Gagne JC. Values clarification exercises to prepare nursing students for artificial intelligence integration. Int J Environ Res Public Health. 2023;20(14):6409.
28. Hoelscher SH, Pugh A. NURSES embracing artificial intelligence: a guide to artificial intelligence literacy for the nursing profession. Nurs Outlook. 2025;73(4):102466.
29. Eden CA, Chisom ON, Adeniyi IS. Integrating AI in education: opportunities, challenges, and ethical considerations. Magna Scientia Adv Res Rev. 2024;10(2):006–13. https://doi.org/10.30574/msarr.2024.10.2.0039.
30. Ibuki T, Ibuki A, Nakazawa E. Possibilities and ethical issues of entrusting nursing tasks to robots and artificial intelligence. Nurs Ethics. 2024;31(6):1010–20. https://doi.org/10.1177/09697330221149094.
31. Konidena BK, Malaiyappan JNA, Tadimarri A. Ethical considerations in the development and deployment of AI systems. Eur J Technol. 2024;8(2):41–53.
32. Al-Hassan M, Dorri R. Harnessing AI for nursing education: innovations, barriers, and ethical considerations. Nurs Educ Innov Ethics. 2025;1:1–11.
33. Molyneux J. Artificial intelligence and nursing: promise and precaution. Am J Nurs. 2023;123(10):17–9. https://doi.org/10.1097/01.NAJ.0000979068.75051.bd. pubmed.ncbi.nlm.nih.gov
34. Wei Q, Pan S, Liu X, Hong M, Nong C, Zhang W. The integration of AI in nursing: addressing current applications, challenges, and future directions. Front Med. 2025;12:1545420.
35. Chu CH, Conway A, Jibb L, Ronquillo CE. The impact of digital technologies, data analytics and AI on nursing informatics: the new skills and knowledge nurses need for the 21st century. In: Delaney CW, Weaver CA, Sensmeier J, Pruinelli L, Weber P, editors. Nursing and informatics for the 21st century—embracing a digital world. 3rd ed. New York, NY: Productivity Press; 2022. p. 149–70. https://doi.org/10.4324/9781003281047. (chapter 9).

Developing AI Literacy for Nurse Leaders and Educators

4

Mary Joy Garcia-Dia

4.1   Introduction

AI is poised to revolutionize healthcare delivery, offering transformative potential across various domains, from enhancing diagnostic accuracy, hybrid models of care, influencing clinical decisions, personalizing treatment plans, improving patient safety to streamlining administrative workflows, and educational tools [1, 2]. However, the efficacy and equity of AI systems are profoundly dependent on the data used for their development and the algorithms that govern their functions. As AI technologies become increasingly integrated into clinical and educational settings, it is imperative that healthcare professionals, particularly nurse leaders and educators develop a mature understanding of these complex systems to demystify the perception of AI as a mysterious "black box" [3]. A thorough understanding of AI, including the complexities of data and algorithms, is vital for nurse leaders to make strategic choices, provide oversight, ensure the ethical deployment of AI, and address any associated risks. Similarly, nurse educators must possess AI literacy in having a deeper comprehension of AI underpinnings and cultivate a foundational understanding of AI technologies and their implications. One has to be competent in navigating the various AI tools and evaluate the appropriate pedagogical content and exercises in teaching AI [4, 5]. To harness these opportunities responsibly, nurse educators must thoughtfully design curricula and structured learning environments, including guiding students to navigate potential risks such as overreliance, misuse, and academic dishonesty [6]. By modeling ethical practices and encouraging reflective co-learning with AI, nurse educators ensure that technology enhances—not replaces—human judgment and professional integrity in nursing education.

M. J. Garcia-Dia (✉)
Nursing, CUNY School of Professional Studies, New York, NY, USA
e-mail: maryjoy.dia@sps.cuny.edu

© The Author(s), under exclusive license to Springer Nature Switzerland AG 2026
D. W. La Rosa et al. (eds.), *Nursing Education in the AI Era*,
https://doi.org/10.1007/978-3-032-12402-9_4

A foundational aspect of AI literacy involves understanding the critical components that drive AI systems: data and algorithms. The quality, representativeness, and integrity of the data fed into AI models, coupled with the design and choices of algorithms, profoundly shape AI's capabilities, outputs, and potential biases [7]. Without this understanding, nurse leaders may struggle to evaluate AI solutions critically, and educators may fail to equip students with the necessary skills to question and validate AI-driven insights.

4.2 The Critical Role of Data in Shaping Artificial Intelligence

Data is the lifeblood of most modern AI systems, particularly those leveraging machine learning (ML) techniques [8]. AI models learn patterns, make predictions, and generate insights based on the data they are trained on. In healthcare, this data can originate from a multitude of sources, including biomedical data sets such as electronic health records (EHRs), medical imaging archives (e.g., X-rays, CT scans, MRIs), genomic sequences, data from wearable sensors, and patient-reported outcomes [9]. The characteristics of this data—its volume, variety, velocity, and veracity—are crucial determinants of an AI model's performance. AI, especially deep learning models, often requires vast amounts of data (big data) to achieve high levels of accuracy and generalizability. Healthcare generates an enormous *volume* of data at high *velocity*, encompassing structured data (e.g., lab values, diagnostic codes, physiological vital signs) and unstructured data (e.g., clinical notes, operative reports, imaging data) [8]. Managing and processing this *variety* and diverse data landscape is very laborious and challenging for humans. Data *veracity* (its accuracy, completeness, consistency, and timeliness) is arguably the most critical factor with AI data to cover the variability of population and sources of meaningful data [9]. The principle of "Garbage In, Garbage Out" (GIGO) is highly pertinent to AI as flawed or poor-quality data will inevitably lead to flawed or unreliable AI outputs [10]. Data preprocessing, which includes cleaning, normalization, transformation, and feature engineering, is a vital, though often overlooked, step in preparing data for AI model training [11].

4.3 The Peril of Bias in Data

Healthcare data is not inherently objective and can reflect historical and systemic biases present in society and clinical practice [7, 12]. If AI models are trained on data that underrepresents certain demographic groups (e.g., based on race, ethnicity, gender, socioeconomic status) or contains biased information, the resulting AI systems can perpetuate and even amplify these biases [13]. For instance, an AI diagnostic tool trained predominantly on data from one demographic might exhibit lower accuracy when applied to other populations, potentially leading to misdiagnosis, health disparities, and inequitable care [12, 14]. Addressing data bias requires careful attention to data collection practices, ensuring dataset diversity, and employing bias detection and mitigation techniques during algorithm design and when training the data [7, 15].

It is essential for nurse leaders and educators to realize that AI tool recommendations are only as reliable as the data used to develop them. Understanding data sources, limitations, and potential for bias is crucial for critically evaluating AI applications.

4.4 Algorithms: The Engine of AI

If data is the fuel, algorithms are the engines of AI systems. An algorithm is a finite sequence of well-defined, computer-implementable instructions, typically to solve a class of problems or to perform a computation [16]. In the context of AI, particularly machine learning, algorithms enable systems to learn from data without being explicitly programmed for each specific task. There are various types of Machine Learning (ML) algorithms, each suited to different kinds of problems:

- *Supervised Learning*: Learns from labeled data to make predictions or classifications [9, 17]. For instance, in nursing, this could involve an AI model trained on electronic health record (EHR) data where patients are labeled as having developed sepsis or not, to predict sepsis risk in new patients. Another example is an algorithm trained on images of various wound types (e.g., pressure injuries, diabetic ulcers), labeled by expert nurses, to classify new wound images and assist in appropriate care planning.
- *Unsupervised Learning*: Identifies patterns in unlabeled data [9, 17]. A nursing-specific use case could be an AI algorithm that analyzes large, complex datasets from wearable sensors and EHRs to identify previously unrecognized patient phenotypes or clusters of patients with similar care needs or responses to nursing interventions, which could inform more personalized care strategies. It might also be used to segment patient populations based on social determinants of health and care utilization patterns to better target community nursing resources and care coordination.
- *Reinforcement Learning*: Learns through trial and error by interacting with the environment and receiving feedback (rewards or penalties) for its actions [9]. In a nursing context, this could be applied to develop AI systems that optimize nurse staffing schedules in real-time based on fluctuating patient acuity and available resources, learning from the impact of past scheduling decisions on patient outcomes and nurse workload. Another example could be an AI-driven education module that adapts its teaching strategy based on a student's engagement and quiz performance, reinforcing learning for better health self-management.

The choice of algorithm, its specific configuration (hyperparameters), and how it is trained significantly influence the AI's output. Different algorithms, even when applied to the same dataset, can yield different predictions or insights. Furthermore, some complex algorithms, like deep neural networks, are often referred to as "black boxes" because their internal decision-making processes can be opaque and difficult for humans to interpret [18]. This lack of transparency can be a barrier to trust and adoption in critical clinical settings, where understanding the rationale behind a decision is paramount [19]. Efforts in "Explainable AI" (XAI) aim to develop techniques that make AI decisions more understandable.

4.5 Critical Concern: Algorithmic Bias

Bias can be introduced not only through data but also through the algorithm's design, the features it prioritizes, or the objective function it is optimized to achieve [7, 14]. As highlighted in Generative AI, training large language models (LLMs) on structured and unstructured datasets enables them to generalize across a wide range of domains [8, 12]. However, this process also carries risks: algorithms may amplify patterns—including biases—present in the data. Moreover, systems like chat GPT (generative pre-trained) transformers depend heavily on vector embeddings which are numeric representations of words, images, phrases, or even entire documents [20]. These numbers are arranged in a way that similar things are close together, like how "doctor" and "nurse" might be near each other because they're related in meaning based on the context of care team. This helps AI systems recognize patterns and make decisions, but if the data used to create these embeddings is biased or incomplete, the system might make unfair or inaccurate assumptions. However, the quality of these embeddings depends on the data they are trained on. If certain concepts or populations are underrepresented or misrepresented in the training data, the resulting vectors may cluster inaccurately, reinforcing stereotypes or omitting critical distinctions. This can lead to biased interpretations and decisions, especially in sensitive domains. An algorithm designed to predict hospital readmission, for example, might inadvertently penalize patients from lower socioeconomic backgrounds if it uses proxies like neighborhood or access to transportation, even if race or income is not explicit [15]. Nurse leaders and educators need a conceptual grasp of how different algorithms work to better understand the strengths, weaknesses, and potential biases of AI tools they encounter or consider for implementation. Other concerns related to AI are access and digital equity. Underrepresented students including those from low-income backgrounds, rural communities, or minoritized racial and linguistic groups, may lack reliable access to AI tools, broadband internet, or devices needed to meaningfully engage with AI-enhanced learning environments [7].

4.6   Building AI Literacy

AI literacy empowers nurses to be informed partners and collaborators in AI implementation, ensuring it enhances patient well-being and upholds the core values of nursing. The American Nurses Association's (ANA) position on artificial intelligence (AI) emphasizes that AI literacy for nurses is crucial for its ethical and effective integration into practice. ANA emphasizes that nurses must understand AI fundamentals, critically evaluate its validity and potential biases, and be keenly aware of ethical implications concerning privacy, autonomy, and equity [21]. AI should augment, not replace, human-centered care, and nurses are accountable for their actions, even when using AI. As nurse leaders, advocating for transparency, educating patients about AI in their care, and committing to continuous learning in this rapidly evolving field is imperative in navigating today's complex digital healthcare environment.

As AI systems become more prevalent, the need for nurses to possess AI literacy—which is the ability to understand, critically evaluate, effectively interact, and utilize AI—becomes increasingly crucial [5, 22]. It encompasses not only technical comprehension but also ethical awareness, data fluency, and decision-making capacity in AI-enhanced environments [5]. Studies have shown that AI offers promising advancements in healthcare which could lead to more efficient patient care and improved decision-making [23]. This highlights the core reason why nurse educators and leaders must prioritize AI literacy and competency in developing collaborative tools to support nursing students' knowledge, clinical skills, and transition to practice.

4.6.1   Foundational Knowledge

AI literacy begins with understanding what AI is and how it functions in healthcare. John McCarthy, in 1955, coined AI's traditional definition as "the science and engineering of making intelligent machines" [24]. The latest definition of AI within healthcare emphasizes its role as a machine-based system capable of analyzing complex medical data to assist and improve patient care, enhance hospital operations, and drive medical innovation [25]. This involves the use of machine learning and other AI techniques to process vast amounts of information, identify patterns, and provide insights for diagnosis, treatment, and administrative efficiency. This includes familiarity with several core AI components described by Beam et al. [26]:

- *Machine learning (ML)*: A method of data analysis that allows computer systems to learn and improve from experience without being explicitly programmed. It is the foundation for many predictive and decision-support tools in healthcare.
- *Natural language processing (NLP)*: A field of AI focused on enabling machines to understand and interpret human language by understanding the structure, grammar, and meaning in words to help computers "understand and compre-

hend" language. Clinical documentation assistants and patient sentiment analysis are powered by NLP.

- *Predictive analytics*: The use of historical data, statistical algorithms, and machine learning to identify the likelihood of future outcomes. It is often used in healthcare to predict patient deterioration, readmission risks, or optimal staffing patterns.
- *Chat-based generative pre-trained transformer (ChatGPT) models*: A system built with a neural network transformer type of AI model that works well in natural language processing tasks. The model (1) can generate responses to questions (*Generative*); (2) was trained in advance on a large amount of the written material available on the web (*Pre-trained*); (3) and can process sentences differently than other types of models (*Transformer*).

4.6.2 Correlating AI Literacy with Roles of Nurse Faculty and Nurse Leaders

Correlating the definition of AI literacy with the roles of nurse faculty and nurse leaders reveals distinct yet interconnected ways AI tools can improve both nursing practice and education:

4.7 AI Literacy for Nurse Faculty

For nurse faculty, AI literacy emphasizes the ability to understand, critically evaluate, and effectively utilize AI technologies in their teaching methodologies and curriculum development. This includes staying current with AI advancements, discerning credible AI resources, and preparing students for an AI-integrated healthcare environment.

- *How AI Tools Improve Education*:
  - *Personalized Learning*: AI-powered learning platforms can analyze student performance data to tailor learning paths, provide targeted feedback, and adapt content to individual learning styles, improving student outcomes [27].
  - *Enhanced Simulation*: AI can enhance the realism and adaptability of virtual reality (VR) and augmented reality (AR) simulations, allowing students to practice clinical skills and decision-making in diverse and complex scenarios without risk to real patients [28, 29].
  - *Automated Assessment and Feedback*: AI tools can automate the grading of assignments, provide immediate feedback on quizzes and exercises, and identify students who may be struggling, allowing faculty to intervene proactively.
  - *Curriculum Development*: AI can assist faculty in identifying current best practices, generating case studies, and updating curriculum content to reflect the evolving role of AI in healthcare [30].

– *AI Literacy Education*: Faculty with strong AI literacy can effectively teach students about AI concepts, ethical considerations, and the responsible use of AI in their future practice [31].

4.8 AI Literacy for Nurse Leaders

For nurse leaders, AI literacy centers on the ability to understand, critically evaluate, and strategically implement and oversee AI solutions to improve patient care, optimize workflows, enhance safety, and promote ethical practices within healthcare organizations. This includes understanding the organizational implications of AI adoption, managing risks, and fostering a culture of innovation [6].

- *How AI Tools Improve Practice*:
    - *Clinical Decision Support*: AI-powered Clinical Decision Support Systems (CDSS) can analyze vast amounts of patient data to provide nurses with evidence-based recommendations, aiding in diagnosis, treatment planning, and early detection of patient deterioration.
    - *Predictive Analytics*: AI can identify patients at high risk for adverse events, such as falls or hospital-acquired infections, allowing for proactive interventions and improved patient safety.
    - *Remote Patient Monitoring*: AI-integrated wearable devices and remote monitoring systems enable nurses to track patient health status remotely, detect subtle changes, and intervene promptly, improving care coordination and access.
    - *Workflow Optimization*: AI can automate administrative tasks, optimize staffing schedules, and prioritize patient needs, reducing nurses' workload and allowing them to focus on direct patient care.
    - *Medication Management*: AI can assist with medication reconciliation, identify potential drug interactions, and improve medication adherence, reducing errors and enhancing patient safety.
    - *Enhanced Communication*: NLP-powered AI can improve communication between nurses, patients, and other healthcare professionals by analyzing patient notes and providing summaries.

The AI literacy of both nurse faculty and nurse leaders is crucial for the successful integration of AI in healthcare. AI-literate faculty can equip future nurses with the foundational knowledge and critical thinking skills to utilize AI tools effectively and ethically in their practice [23]. Simultaneously, AI-literate nurse leaders can champion the responsible adoption of AI within healthcare organizations, ensuring that these technologies are implemented in a way that enhances patient care, supports nursing staff, and aligns with ethical and regulatory standards [6, 32]. Furthermore, AI-literate leaders can support faculty development in AI literacy, recognizing that well-prepared educators are essential for cultivating an AI-ready nursing workforce [33]. This creates a positive feedback loop where knowledgeable leaders empower educators, who in turn empower future practitioners, leading to a healthcare system that can leverage the full potential of AI for improved patient outcomes and a more efficient and effective nursing profession.

4.8.1 Essential Competencies for Critical Appraisal of AI Tools

AI software, both commercial and open source, offers numerous options. For example, a query using an advanced AI model like Google Gemini Advanced [34] on AI systems and software applications used or with potential use in healthcare can generate a plethora of products (see Appendix A). Being familiar with AI products' functions and features can initially provide nurse educators with informed choices in identifying which products or AI concepts have the most meaningful use in teaching and preparing future nurses to critically assess the impact of AI tools and their ethical implementation in education and practice (see Appendix A). For example, virtual assistants can assist educators in drafting lectures and tutorial content, personalizing learning guides, finding visual representations of content, and designing lesson plans and assessments.

Nurse educators require distinct competencies to effectively integrate AI into curricula and guide learners in a digitally transforming healthcare environment. Leveraging interdisciplinary frameworks from the World Health Organization's guidance on digital health competencies, recommendations from the International Medical Informatics Association, and pedagogical models such as the PAIR framework and AI in Learning competency matrix [32, 35], these competencies include:

- *Digital Pedagogy*: The ability to integrate AI tools into active, student-centered learning designs, including simulation, gamification, and flipped classroom models [4].
- *Ethical Reasoning in AI Contexts*: Educators must evaluate and teach about bias, consent, privacy, and data justice embedded in AI tools [7, 12].
- *AI Fluency*: A working knowledge of large language models (LLMs), natural language processing (NLP), and machine learning is essential to make informed decisions about using AI-enhanced assessments and feedback [19].
- *Critical Evaluation of AI Content*: The skill to appraise AI-generated content for accuracy, relevance, and pedagogical value is necessary to prevent the dissemination of misinformation or overreliance [4].
- *Change Leadership*: Educators must lead cultural shifts in academic settings that promote critical digital literacy, institutional policy alignment, and collaborative innovation in AI adoption [32].

These sources emphasize that critical AI appraisal requires not only technical understanding but also ethical reasoning, cultural awareness, and reflective practice. These competencies ensure that nurse educators remain not only effective facilitators of student learning, but also ethical stewards of emerging technologies.

4.9 Integrating AI in Nursing Education: Competencies, Challenges, and Strategic Imperatives

The integration of artificial intelligence (AI) into nursing education—through tools such as AI-powered learning platforms, simulation technologies, clinical decision support systems (CDSS), and virtual assistants—offers significant potential to support student nurses as they transition into clinical practice [28]. However, realizing this potential requires intentional strategies and clearly defined competencies for both nurse educators and nurse leaders.

4.9.1 Scenario for Nurse Educators: Facilitating AI-Enhanced Learning

Nurse educators are pivotal in designing learning experiences that prepare students to critically engage with AI tools. For example, educators can incorporate AI-driven simulations that present dynamic, lifelike patient scenarios. These simulations allow students to practice clinical reasoning, interpret AI-generated recommendations, and apply ethical decision-making in a safe environment [27]. Through this process, students build confidence, develop clinical judgment, and learn to integrate CDSS into their workflow to support diagnosis, treatment planning, and early detection of patient deterioration.

To succeed in this role, nurse educators must demonstrate competencies in:

- *Digital and AI literacy*: Understanding how AI tools function and how to teach their application.
- *Curriculum design*: Embedding AI ethics, equity, and critical thinking into learning modules.
- *Simulation and experiential learning*: Using immersive technologies to replicate real-world clinical challenges.
- *Ethical facilitation*: Guiding students in navigating data privacy, bias, and responsible AI use.

4.9.2 Scenario for Nurse Leaders: Guiding Ethical AI Integration in Practice

As new nurses transition into practice and grow into leadership roles, their early exposure to AI tools equips them to influence how these technologies are implemented and governed. Nurse leaders can advocate for the ethical use of AI, ensuring that tools are equitable, transparent, and aligned with patient-centered care [20, 21]. For instance, a nurse leader might lead an initiative to evaluate the fairness of a predictive algorithm used in patient triage, asking critical questions such as the following: *What data was this AI trained on? Is it representative of our patient population? What are its limitations?*

Key competencies for nurse leaders include:

- *AI governance and policy development*—nurse leaders must be equipped in establishing structure and governance to guide institutional policies with the use of AI tools that includes data privacy, testing and downtime processes.
- *Interdisciplinary collaboration with data scientists and ethicists*—Nurse leaders must be able to communicate clinical needs and ethical concerns to technical teams. Through a collaboration, nurses can lead in co-designing machine learning models like sepsis detection, ensuring it aligns with clinical workflows.
- *Strategic planning for AI adoption and training*—readiness assessment and customizing training programs based on user role is critical in the safe adoption of AI tools.
- *Oversight of AI performance, safety, and equity*—mechanisms that evaluate outcomes, track AI performance and address unintended consequences will ensure trust and confidence in the use of reliable AI tools.

4.10 Challenges and Strategic Imperatives

Several challenges hinder the widespread development of AI literacy within nursing. Nurses exhibit varying levels of comfort and confidence with emerging technologies, which can lead to hesitation or resistance in adopting AI tools. The demanding academic schedules and competing clinical priorities prevent nurses to find the time to engage in additional training, especially within an already stressful environment. Compounding this issue is the rapid pace of technological advancement, which can render newly acquired knowledge obsolete in a short period. Additionally, there is a scarcity of nursing-specific AI educational resources that are both accessible and relevant to the unique contexts of nursing practice. Addressing these challenges requires intentional strategies that support ongoing learning, build confidence, and ensure that AI education is tailored to the realities of nursing roles. To address these barriers, the following strategic imperatives are essential:

1. *Tailored AI Literacy Programs*: Develop nursing-specific training that includes modules on ethics, equity, and real-world application [3, 6, 35].
2. *Interdisciplinary Collaboration*: Engage experts from nursing, informatics, data science, and bioethics to co-create relevant educational content.
3. *Practical Resources*: Provide toolkits, case studies, and frameworks to support responsible AI use [36].
4. *Lifelong Learning Culture*: Promote continuous professional development to keep pace with evolving AI technologies [32].
5. *Research and Evidence Building*: Invest in studies that evaluate the impact of AI on nursing practice, patient outcomes, and health equity as well as AI literacy interventions addressing bias and promoting fairness [15, 37].

4.10.1 Utilizing Scenario-Based Learning (SBL) and Case Studies to Navigate Equity Barriers

As AI becomes increasingly embedded in care delivery and education, leaders must combine clinical reasoning, digital fluency, and ethical vigilance. To effectively prepare nursing students to navigate the complex ethical landscape of AI in healthcare, particularly concerning equity, educators can leverage pedagogical strategies such as scenario-based learning (SBL) and case studies [38]. These methods foster critical thinking, ethical reasoning, and the application of knowledge to real-world or simulated situations where AI intersects with patient care and potential health disparities [37, 39].

Nurse leaders can assess AI tools with the same rigor as clinical research when evaluating credibility. This includes scrutinizing sources and design of AI tools, analyzing validation studies, comparing performance metrics and examining funding sources and conflict of interest. To support the integration of these strategies, nurse educators can access a growing body of resources, including open-access repositories of AI-related case studies, simulation platforms that incorporate generative AI, and professional development modules offered by organizations such as the American Association of Colleges of Nursing (AACN), the National League for Nursing (NLN), and the Alliance for Nursing Informatics. These resources provide practical tools for embedding AI ethics and equity into curricula, including templates for scenario creation, guides for evaluating AI tools, and frameworks for inclusive teaching practices. For example, educators can also explore NLN's Teaching Resources hub, which includes equitable and inclusive toolkits, virtual simulations, and scenario templates that can be adapted to include AI-related dilemmas. These resources empower faculty to embed AI ethics and equity into curricula with confidence and creativity.

However, the promise of AI in nursing education and practice is tempered by significant equity concerns. Equity barriers in AI can manifest in various ways within nursing student learning and clinical practice. These include algorithmic bias stemming from unrepresentative training data. AI systems trained on homogenous datasets may reflect the dominant demographic, marginalizing those with different cultural, linguistic, or educational contexts. Studies show that AI-generated patient education content, such as ChatGPT-4 responses, are written at a high reading level, averaging grade 11 or higher, which exceeds the recommended sixth grade reading level for health materials [12, 15]. This readability barrier can exclude learners with limited literacy or English as a second language. If these tools are embedded into assessment or feedback mechanisms, they may penalize students who diverge from the norm as well as lead to poorer outcomes for marginalized populations [12, 15, 40]; disparities in access to AI tools and the digital literacy required to use them effectively among both patients and providers [34, 41]; and the potential for AI to inadvertently reinforce existing societal biases if not critically evaluated [7].

Scenario-based learning allows students to engage in complex, realistic situations where AI is a component of care. For instance, generative AI can be used to create intricate ethical dilemmas related to AI, such as diagnostic AI providing recommendations that seem to conflict with a patient's expressed cultural values or socioeconomic realities [40]. Students working in groups can analyze these scenarios, propose solutions, and debate the ethical implications of different actions, thereby enhancing their understanding of how AI outputs must be contextualized with patient-specific factors and a commitment to equity [41]. Role-playing within these scenarios where students might take on roles of the nurse, patient, AI developer, or ethicist can further deepen empathy and appreciation for diverse perspectives [40].

Case studies, particularly those drawn from real-world instances of AI application or well-constructed hypothetical examples, are powerful tools for illustrating the tangible impacts of AI on health equity. Analyzing cases where AI either exacerbated or helped mitigate health disparities can provide profound learning opportunities. For example, discussing the case of pulse oximeter inaccuracies in patients with darker skin tones due to biased sensor development [42], or an algorithm that incorrectly flagged certain patient populations as lower risk due to socioeconomic proxies in the data [12], can make the concept of algorithmic bias concrete. Educators can guide students to dissect these cases, identify the points at which bias was introduced or could have been challenged, and explore strategies for developing and deploying AI more equitably. Furthermore, AI itself can be used to develop unfolding case studies, allowing for dynamic learning experiences where students make decisions and see the consequences in a simulated environment [30, 43].

These active learning strategies encourage both faculty and students to move beyond theoretical knowledge to practical application, fostering skills in:

- *Critical Appraisal*: Evaluating AI tool outputs for potential bias and relevance to diverse patient populations.
- *Ethical Decision-Making*: Navigating dilemmas where AI recommendations may conflict with equitable care principles.
- *Advocacy*: Championing the fair and just use of AI and advocating for patients who may be negatively impacted by biased systems.
- *Communication*: Discussing AI's role and limitations with patients and interprofessional teams, ensuring transparency and shared understanding.

By integrating SBL and case studies focused on AI and equity into nursing curricula, educators can better prepare future nurses to be vigilant guardians against AI-induced health disparities and proactive agents in harnessing AI to promote health equity for all [3, 36]. This includes fostering an understanding of how to involve diverse patient communities in the design and testing of AI tools to prevent bias from the outset [42, 44].

4.10.2 Evaluating AI Solutions in Real Patient Care Scenarios

Evaluating AI solutions in real patient care scenarios requires a rigorous and multifaceted approach. Frameworks like those promoted by the Agency for Healthcare

Research and Quality (AHRQ) for patient safety and quality research, and the National Institute of Standards and Technology (NIST) AI Risk Management Framework (AI RMF) offer valuable lenses through which to analyze and assess these technologies [45, 46].

1. *Agency for Healthcare Research and Quality (AHRQ) Patient Safety and Quality Principles*

While AHRQ may not have a singular framework for AI evaluation, its broader work and the principles of patient safety and quality research design it promotes are highly relevant. AHRQ focuses on improving the safety and quality of healthcare through research and evidence-based practice. Key concepts from AHRQ's approach that can be applied to evaluating AI in patient care include the Six Domains of Healthcare Quality (originally from the Institute of Medicine, now National Academy of Medicine): safety, effectiveness, patient-centeredness, timeliness, efficiency, and equity [45]. These domains provide a comprehensive structure for evaluating any healthcare intervention, including AI. A core principle is preventing harm, emphasizing implementation context, and the importance of measuring impact on patient outcomes and quality metrics.

- *Analysis for Evaluating AI in Real Patient Care*: Applying AHRQ's principles and the IOM's six domains can help evaluate AI solutions by assessing:
  - *Safety*: Risk assessment for new hazards, mitigation strategies, and transparency for clinicians.
  - *Effectiveness*: Clinical validation of improved outcomes, appropriate use, and avoidance of misuse.
  - *Patient-Centeredness*: Consideration of patient values, impact on patient experience, communication, and trust.
  - *Timeliness*: Impact on workflow speed and efficiency without compromising quality.
  - *Efficiency*: Optimization of resource utilization and cost-effectiveness.
  - *Equity*: Rigorous testing for biases and ensuring fair access for all patient populations.

2. *AI Risk Management Framework (NIST AI RMF)*

The NIST AI Risk Management Framework (AI RMF) is a comprehensive guide for organizations to manage risks associated with AI systems throughout their lifecycle. It provides a structured approach to identify, assess, and mitigate AI risks while promoting trustworthiness and responsible AI development and use. The AI RMF is built around four core functions: Govern, Map, Measure, and Manage [46]. It also emphasizes characteristics of trustworthy AI: valid and reliable; safe; secure and resilient; accountable and transparent; explainable and interpretable; privacy-enhanced; and fair with harmful bias mitigated. Academic medical institutions and healthcare organizations can leverage this framework in promoting trust through a robust governance structure ensuring that there is a human in the loop in evaluating AI risks.

Both the principles embedded in AHRQ's work on patient safety and quality and the structured approach of the NIST AI Risk Management Framework provide essential guidance for evaluating AI solutions in real patient care. A comprehensive evaluation should consider the clinical context, potential risks and benefits across the domains of healthcare quality, and the trustworthiness of the AI system throughout its lifecycle. By applying these frameworks, healthcare organizations can make more informed decisions about adopting AI technologies that are safe, effective, patient-centered, and equitable. It is crucial to move beyond solely technical evaluations and incorporate these broader perspectives, including pedagogical strategies like scenario-based learning and case studies to address equity, to ensure responsible and beneficial integration of AI into clinical practice. Ultimately, developing AI literacy among nurse educators and leaders is not merely a matter of technological proficiency. It is a fundamental requirement for ensuring that AI serves to enhance, rather than compromise, the core values of nursing: patient-centered care, safety, ethics, and justice [6, 32].

4.11　Conclusion

The integration of artificial intelligence (AI) into nursing education and practice marks a pivotal moment in the evolution of the profession. AI tools ranging from clinical decision support systems to intelligent simulation platforms offer transformative opportunities to enhance learning, improve patient outcomes, and promote health equity. However, the successful adoption of these technologies depends on the readiness of nurse educators and leaders to guide the next generation of nurses through this transition.

Data and algorithms are the foundational pillars upon which AI systems are built. Their characteristics, quality, and design profoundly influence the performance, reliability, and fairness of AI applications in healthcare [46]. For nurse leaders and educators, a robust understanding of these elements is not merely a technical requirement but a professional and ethical imperative. AI literacy, cultivated through targeted education that includes strategies like scenario-based learning and case studies, and guided by evaluation frameworks such as those from AHRQ and NIST [21, 45, 46], empowers nurse leaders to guide their organizations through the complexities of AI adoption. It enables nurse educators to prepare a new generation of nurses who are not only skilled in using AI tools but are also critical thinkers capable of safeguarding patient interests and promoting health equity in an AI-augmented healthcare landscape [47, 48].

By demystifying AI and fostering a deeper understanding of its core components and societal implications, the nursing profession can harness the immense potential of AI to improve patient care, enhance operational efficiency, and advance health equity—while proactively mitigating its inherent risks [49]. The journey toward comprehensive AI literacy in nursing requires a concerted and ongoing commitment from individuals, educational institutions, healthcare organizations, and professional bodies [31, 50].

The future of AI in nursing is promising. Intelligent tutoring systems could personalize education based on individual learning styles. Virtual patients may evolve in real time based on student decisions, offering deeper experiential learning. Predictive analytics could help nurses anticipate patient needs before symptoms arise [51]. These innovations not only enhance clinical preparedness but also reduce cognitive burden and support safer, more efficient care delivery.

As we embrace this future, it is essential to preserve the core values of nursing—empathy, holistic assessment, and critical thinking. AI should serve as a complement to the human touch, not a replacement. With strategic preparation, nurse educators and leaders can ensure that the next generation of nurses is equipped to thrive in a digitally enhanced healthcare environment and to lead the ethical, equitable, and effective integration of AI across the continuum of human-centered care.

Appendix A: Commercial AI Product

Nursing, health education and learning tools	Description
Sherpath AI	Faculty lesson planning and active learning
GoodNurse	Personalized study plans for nursing students
Mindgrasp AI	Summarizes and quizzes from learning materials
AlertWatch OB	Maternal care alerts
AITRICS VitalCare	Predictive analytics from EHR
Remote monitoring and patient care	
Vitalera	Remote patient monitoring using AI
AITRICS VitalCare	Predicts patient deterioration using EHR data
AlertWatch OB	Maternal surveillance system with real-time alerts during labor and delivery
Amwell Converge	Digital healthcare platform with AI-powered virtual nursing
LookDeep Health	AI and computer vision for real-time patient behavior insights
Teton	AI-powered caregiving system using optical sensors
Conversational and general AI assistants	
ChatGPT (OpenAI)	Conversational AI for dialogue, reasoning, and content generation
Claude (Anthropic)	Focused on dialogue, summarization, and complex reasoning
Copilot (Microsoft)	Integrated AI assistant in Microsoft products
Duet AI (Google)	AI assistant for Google Workspace and Cloud
Einstein (Salesforce)	AI assistant in CRM tools
IBM Watson	AI for customer service, employee Q&A, and coding assistance

(continued)

Enterprise and productivity AI	
Copilot *(Microsoft)*	AI in Microsoft 365 and other tools
Duet AI *(Google)*	AI in Google Workspace
Einstein *(Salesforce)*	CRM AI assistant
SAP Business AI	Embedded AI in SAP products
Dell AI Solutions	AI for data insights and productivity
NVIDIA AI Platform	Cloud-based AI software platform
IBM Watson	AI for enterprise Q&A and automation
Customer service and relationship management	
Kustomer	AI-powered customer service software
Clay	AI for relationship ecosystem management
Grammarly	AI writing assistant

This appendix presents a representative sample of commercially available AI products solely for educational and illustrative purposes. The list is not comprehensive of all products in the marketplace and should not be interpreted as an endorsement or recommendation of any specific product.

References

1. Al Kuwaiti A, Nazer K, Al-Reedy A, Al-Shehri S, Al-Muhanna A, Vijay A, et al. A review of the role of artificial intelligence in healthcare. J Pers Med. 2023;13(6):951. https://doi.org/10.3390/jpm13060951.
2. De Micco F, Di Palma G, Ferorelli D, De Benedictis A, Tomassini L, Tambone V. Artificial intelligence in healthcare: transforming patient safety with intelligent systems: a systematic review. Front Med. 2025;11:1522554. Available from: https://www.frontiersin.org/journals/medicine/articles/10.3389/fmed.2024.1522554/full.
3. El Arab R, Al Moosa O, Abuadas F, Somerville J. The role of AI in nursing education and practice: umbrella review. J Med Internet Res. 2025;27:e69881. https://www.jmir.org/2025/1/e69881. Accessed 9th May 2025.
4. Niemi H, Pea RD, Lu Y, editors. AI in learning: designing the future. Cham: Springer Nature; 2023. https://doi.org/10.1007/978-3-031-09687-7.
5. Arjanto P. Harnessing artificial intelligence: transformational leadership and ethical integration in nursing education and practice. Teach Learn Nurs. 2025. https://doi.org/10.1016/j.teln.2025.01.032.
6. Dorin M, Atkinson HL. Getting to know AI; gaps and opportunities for nurse educators. Teach Learn Nurs. 2024;19(3):218–24. https://doi.org/10.1016/j.teln.2024.02.013.
7. Norori N, Hu Q, Aellen FM, Faraci FD, Tzovara A. Addressing bias in big data and AI for health care: a call for open science. Patterns (NY). 2021;2(10):100347. https://doi.org/10.1016/j.patter.2021.100347.
8. Davenport T, Kalakota R. The potential for artificial intelligence in healthcare. Future Healthc J. 2019;6(2):94–8. https://doi.org/10.7861/futurehosp.6-2-94.
9. Pereira T, Morgado J, Silva F, Pelter MM, Dias VR, Barros R, et al. Sharing biomedical data: strengthening AI development in healthcare. Healthcare (Basel). 2021;9(7):827. https://doi.org/10.3390/healthcare9070827.
10. Pantielieiev D. Garbage in, garbage out: how to stop your AI from hallucinating. Shelf.io. 2025. Available from: https://shelf.io/blog/garbage-in-garbage-out-ai-implementation/.
11. Chicco D, Rovelli C. Eleven quick tips for data cleaning and feature engineering. PLoS Comput Biol. 2022;18(12):e1010747. https://doi.org/10.1371/journal.pcbi.1010718.

12. Obermeyer Z, Powers B, Vogeli C, Mullainathan S. Dissecting racial bias in an algorithm used to manage the health of populations. Science. 2019;366(6464):447–53. https://doi.org/10.1126/science.aax2342.
13. Wiens J, Saria S, Sendak M, Ghassemi M, Liu VX, Doshi-Velez F, et al. Do no harm: a roadmap for responsible machine learning for health care. Nat Med. 2019;25(9):1337–40. https://doi.org/10.1038/s41591-019-0609-x.
14. Rajkomar A, Dean J, Kohane I. Machine learning in medicine. N Engl J Med. 2019;380(14):1347–58.
15. Cary MP Jr. School of Nursing Faculty and Inaugural AI Health Equity Scholar aims to eliminate algorithmic bias in healthcare. Duke University School of Nursing News. 2023. Available from: https://nursing.duke.edu/news/ai-health-equity-scholar-works-against-bias.
16. Obermeyer Z, Emanuel EJ. Predicting the future: big data, machine learning, and clinical medicine. N Engl J Med. 2016;375(13):1216–9. https://doi.org/10.1056/NEJMp1606181.
17. An Q, Rahman S, Zhou J, Kang JJ. A comprehensive review on machine learning in healthcare industry: classification, restrictions, opportunities and challenges. Sensors (Basel). 2023;23(9):4178. https://doi.org/10.3390/s23094178.
18. Adadi A, Berrada M. Peeking inside the black-box: a survey on explainable artificial intelligence (XAI). IEEE Access. 2018;6:52138–60.
19. Tonekaboni S, Joshi S, McCradden MD, Goldenberg A. What Clinicians want: contextualizing explainable machine learning for clinical end use. In: Proceedings of the 4th machine learning for healthcare conference in proceedings of machine learning research, vol 106; 2019. p. 359–80 Available from https://proceedings.mlr.press/v106/tonekaboni19a.html.
20. Syed HF. How AI learns hidden patterns: the power of embeddings in predictions. Int J Sci Technol. 2025;16(1):45–58. https://doi.org/10.71097/IJSAT.v16.i1.2596.
21. American Nurses Association. The ethical use of artificial intelligence in nursing practice [Internet]. Silver Spring: ANA; 2022 [cited 2025 May 11]. Available from: https://www.nursingworld.org/globalassets/practiceandpolicy/nursing-excellence/ana-position-statements/the-ethical-use-of-artificial-intelligence-in-nursing-practice_bod-approved-12_20_22.pdf.
22. Nurse.com. The ethical implications of AI in nursing [Internet]. Nurse.com. 2024 [cited 2025 May 10]. Available from: https://www.nurse.com/blog/ethical-implications-ai-nursing-nsp/.
23. McGowan S, Bolster N, Rutledge G. Artificial intelligence in nursing education: a scoping review. Nurse Educ Pract. 2021;54:103131.
24. McCarthy J. What is AI? [Internet]. Stanford University [cited 2025 May 10]. Available from: http://jmc.stanford.edu/artificial-intelligence/what-is-ai/.
25. Congressional Research Service. Artificial Intelligence (AI) in health care. Report R48319 [Internet]. Washington, DC: Congress.gov [cited 2025 May 10]. Available from: https://www.congress.gov/crs-product/R48319.
26. Beam AL, Kohane IS. Big data and machine learning in health care. JAMA. 2018;319(13):1317–8.
27. Hwang GJ, Xie HC, Zeng QH, Abelson S. Applying artificial intelligence to enhance learning in STEM education: a review. Comput Educ Artif Intell. 2021;2:100027.
28. Radianti J, Majchrzak TA, Fromm J, Wohlgenannt I. A systematic review of immersive virtual reality applications for higher education: design elements, lessons learned, and research agenda. Comput Educ. 2020;147:103778. https://doi.org/10.1016/j.compedu.2019.103778.
29. Gibson G, Gandomkar Z, Ebrahimi S. The impact of artificial intelligence on nursing students: a systematic review. ResearchGate. 2025 [Preprint]. Available from: https://www.researchgate.net/publication/389097107_The_Impact_of_Artificial_Intelligence_on_Nursing_Students_A_Systematic_Review.
30. Silvestri-Elmore A, Burton C. How can nursing faculty create case studies using AI and educational technology? Nurse Educ. 2025;50(1):35–9. https://doi.org/10.1097/NNE.0000000000001734.
31. Simms R. Generative artificial intelligence (AI) literacy in nursing education: a crucial call to action. Nurse Educ Today. 2025;146:106544.
32. World Health Organization. Ethics and governance of artificial intelligence for health. Geneva: WHO; 2021.

33. Kotp MH, Ismail HA, Basyouny HAA, Aly MA, Hendy A, Nashwan AJ, et al. Empowering nurse leaders: readiness for AI integration and the perceived benefits of predictive analytics. BMC Nurs. 2025;24:56. https://doi.org/10.1186/s12912-024-02653-x.
34. Google. Gemini advanced [Large language model]. 2025 [cited 2025 May 11]. Available from: https://gemini.google.com/advanced.
35. Chee H, Ahn S, Lee J. A competency framework for AI literacy: variations by different learner groups and an implied learning pathway. Br J Educ Technol. 2024:1–37. https://doi.org/10.1111/bjet.13556.
36. Morin A. Why nurse leaders deserve a seat at the AI table. HIT Consultant. 2025 [cited 2025 May 10]. Available from: https://hitconsultant.net/2025/04/03/why-nurse-leaders-deserve-a-seat-at-the-ai-table/.
37. Sadeghi M, Nematollahi M, Farokhzadian J, Khoshnood Z, Eghbalian M. The effect of scenario-based training on the Core competencies of nursing students: a semi-experimental study. BMC Nurs. 2023;22(1):475. https://doi.org/10.1186/s12912-023-01442-2.
38. Zheng K, Shen Z, Chen Z, Che C, Zhu H. Application of AI-empowered scenario-based simulation teaching mode in cardiovascular disease education. BMC Med Educ. 2024;24:1003. https://doi.org/10.1186/s12909-024-05977-z.
39. Morley J, Machado CC, Burr C, Cowls J, Joshi I, Taddeo M, Floridi L. The ethics of AI in health care: a mapping review. Soc Sci Med. 2020;260:113172.
40. Al-Hassan M, Dorri R. Harnessing AI for nursing education: innovations, barriers, and ethical considerations. ARV J. 2025;1(1):1–11.
41. Center for Teaching and Learning, Northern Michigan University. Exploring critical thinking and ethics with generative AI. NMU CTL Resources. Available from: https://nmu.edu/ctl/exploring-critical-thinking-and-ethics. Accessed 11 May 2025.
42. Stetler C. AI algorithms used in healthcare can perpetuate bias. Rutgers University-Newark News. 2024. Available from: https://www.newark.rutgers.edu/news/ai-algorithms-used-healthcare-can-perpetuate-bias.
43. Harvard Medical School Postgraduate Education. AI implications for health equity: Shaping the future of healthcare quality and safety. Harvard Medical School Postgraduate Education Trends in Medicine. 2025. Available from: https://postgraduateeducation.hms.harvard.edu/trends-medicine/ai-implications-health-equity-shaping-future-health-care-quality-safety.
44. Shen M, Shen Y, Liu F, Jin J. Prompts, privacy, and personalized learning: integrating AI into nursing education: a qualitative study. BMC Nurs. 2025;24:470. https://doi.org/10.1186/s12912-025-03115-8.
45. Shenoy A. Patient safety from the perspective of quality management frameworks: a review. Patient Saf Surg. 2021;15(1):12. https://doi.org/10.1186/s13037-021-00286-6.
46. Raimondo GM, Lacascio LE. Artificial intelligence risk management framework. National Institute of Standards and Technology U.S. Department of Commerce; 2023. https://doi.org/10.6028/NIST.AI.100-1.
47. Ronquillo CE, Peltonen LM, Pruinelli L, Chu CH, Bakken S, Beduschi A, et al. Artificial intelligence in nursing: priorities and opportunities from an international invitational think-tank of the nursing and artificial intelligence leadership collaborative. J Adv Nurs. 2021;77(9):3707–17. https://doi.org/10.1111/jan.14855.
48. Kong G, Liu J, Lu S, Liu M, Meng L. Generative artificial intelligence (AI) literacy in nursing education: a crucial call to action. Nurse Educ Today. 2025;148:106553.
49. Kumar P, Chauhan S, Awasthi LK. Artificial intelligence in healthcare; review, ethics, trust challenges and future research directions. Eng Appl Artif Intell. 2023;120:105894. https://doi.org/10.1016/j.engappai.2023.105894.
50. Topol EJ. High-performance medicine: the convergence of human and artificial intelligence. Nat Med. 2019;25(1):44–56.
51. Ahmed SK. Artificial intelligence in nursing: current trends, possibilities and pitfalls. J Med Surg Public Health. 2024;3:100072. https://doi.org/10.1016/j.glmedi.2024.100072.

Integrating AI into the Nursing Curriculum

5

Delaney Wright La Rosa and Jennifer Adrian Rossetti

5.1   Introduction: A New Landscape for Nursing Education

Artificial intelligence (AI) is no longer emerging in nursing education; it is embedded, evolving, and, at times, erupting into headlines with both promise and controversy. As clinical and educational environments increasingly rely on sophisticated technologies and AI-supported tools, the competencies needed by future nurses are shifting [1, 2]. To meet this challenge, teaching must evolve, not simply to incorporate new tools, but to cultivate an ethos of digitally enhanced learning and AI-supported growth. Nurse educators have a unique opportunity to lead this shift, shaping the future of AI-integrated learning environments with intentionality and learner-centered design. Future educators will prepare students not only to deliver patient-centered care but also to collaborate effectively with technology as a routine aspect of clinical practice [3, 4].

This chapter invites nurse educators to explore how AI can enhance and expand teaching and learning. Rather than presenting AI as a one-size-fits-all solution, the chapter frames AI as a flexible teaching partner, one that can be integrated with existing pedagogical goals to create more inclusive, responsive, and competency-aligned learning environments [5–7]. Tools and strategies that support cognitive, affective, and psychomotor learning, using real-world examples and practical steps that educators can adapt based on their course goals and student needs, are

D. W. La Rosa (✉)
Florida State University College of Nursing, Tallahassee, FL, USA
e-mail: DWLaRosa@fsu.edu

J. A. Rossetti
College of Nursing, Northern Arizona University, Flagstaff, AZ, USA
e-mail: Jennifer.Rossetti@nau.edu

D. W. La Rosa et al. (eds.), *Nursing Education in the AI Era*,
https://doi.org/10.1007/978-3-032-12402-9_5

highlighted. Most importantly, educators should read this chapter through the lens that they *need not become AI experts*. Instead, educators should lean into a clear understanding of what students must learn while adding a curiosity and willingness to experiment with tools that have the potential to accelerate knowledge acquisition.

5.2 Designing with AI for Knowledge Mastery

Students historically find courses like pharmacology challenging [8, 9]. Educators may notice students struggling to retain content, apply it consistently, and build confidence over time. Despite educators' best efforts, review sessions, practice quizzes, and office hours, the diversity in how students learn and what they retain can leave significant gaps. These gaps are not necessarily due to a failure to learn [10, 11]. More often, they reflect the complexity of nursing content and the wide variability in learners' backgrounds, cognitive styles, prior knowledge, and even stress levels [12]. Traditionally, educators have tried to meet these needs with static interventions such as textbook problem sets or generalized tutoring recommendations, yet these approaches may fall short of adapting to each student's evolving understanding [13, 14].

Persistent gaps like these are an excellent example of where AI can extend the educator's role. Adaptive learning tools, powered by artificial intelligence, allow educators to create more personalized learning pathways and extend their presence beyond the classroom [5, 14]. Platforms such as StudyFetch, Quizlet AI, OpenAI's Study Mode, and MagicSchool now allow both educators and students to convert lecture materials into individualized study supports, often at the touch of a button [15–17]. Students can upload class notes, slide decks, and readings to generate personalized flashcards, quizzes, narrated summaries, or even visual concept maps. These tools adjust content based on performance, promoting spaced repetition and deeper processing. In short, they help students study the right material at the right time, in a format that meets their learning needs [3, 13].

Imagine a student entering the second week of pathophysiology, overwhelmed by new terminology and complex mechanisms. They upload their notes to an adaptive platform, which then creates a podcast or short video summarizing the key concepts they marked as confusing. As they review, the platform tracks their performance and gradually increases complexity. Meanwhile, the educator can access anonymized, aggregate data highlighting common areas of misunderstanding. This insight informs upcoming lectures, helps shape in-class examples, and supports targeted formative assessment. Even minimal use of AI tools in this way can enhance both learner autonomy and instructional precision.

Getting started with AI-supported tools doesn't require a full course redesign or specialized informational technology (IT) integration. Many adaptive platforms are designed for ease of use; students can access them independently, and educators can integrate them into their teaching with little more than a link or assignment suggestion. In fact, 50% of college students say that they currently use AI tools such as these on their own [18]. Educators who take time to explore how students are studying may discover that learners are uploading lecture slides, generating summaries or flashcards, and using AI-generated questions to guide reviews. Recognizing and engaging with these informal learning practices allows educators to better understand how students are interacting with course content and to offer guidance that aligns student effort with instructional goals. Even modest utilization can help ensure that AI becomes a bridge between educator intention and student learning.

Why are students using platforms such as StudyFetch and Quizlet AI? The answer is simple: the experience is customized, adaptive, and engaging [15, 16, 18, 19]. When students upload content, platforms can instantly generate study materials in formats such as podcasts, flashcards, quizzes, timelines, videos, or chatbot-style explanations [15–17]. Students can listen to narrated summaries while commuting, use visual mapping tools to study for exams, or quiz themselves with material tailored to their strengths and weaknesses. As students continue to engage, the system adjusts in real time, providing additional support where needed and moving more quickly through mastered topics. For learners balancing multiple responsibilities, learning in a second language, or navigating neurodivergence, this kind of responsive, multimodal engagement can significantly improve self-efficacy and persistence [13, 18, 19].

Scenario A nursing educator is exploring the possibility of adopting an institution-wide adaptive learning platform (like StudyFetch, Quizlet AI, or MagicSchool). Initially, the educator might be concerned about what students could upload to the platform. However, they quickly discover that students are already using these tools independently, often uploading instructor-provided materials. This opens up the potential for violation of copyright law, as it constitutes the unauthorized distribution of intellectual property owned by the educator and/or the academic institution. Partnering with the college's IT department, the team is able to negotiate an institutional license that gives educators control over uploaded content while preserving privacy and delivering actionable learning data. Instructors are then able to focus on curating high-quality materials for upload and preparing weekly plans that utilize platform reports highlighting student learning needs. Student engagement increases, and educators have real-time data informing them about their students' strengths and weaknesses.

AI-supported adaptive learning platforms, however, should not be treated as passive content generators. Educator guidance is essential. Educators should help students critically evaluate AI-generated content, validate answers against course objectives, and use AI tools to supplement, not replace, intentional study. When integrated with purpose, adaptive platforms become a pedagogical scaffold. They promote retrieval practice, adjust to pacing needs, and surface gaps in understanding. This learning approach mirrors the foundational principles of both Bloom's revised taxonomy and Universal Design for Learning (UDL) [20–22]. AI tools can provide differentiated pathways without sacrificing rigor and support more equitable learning experiences across a range of learner needs and contexts. When used intentionally and ethically, adaptive AI can promote not just content mastery but deeper cognitive engagement and inclusivity, but is not without risks [19, 22].

From a pedagogical standpoint, the independent use of AI tools presents several risks to a student's cognitive growth. AI tools are designed to provide answers and summaries, which prevent students from wrestling with complex topics, crucial for deep, long-term learning. This risks students learning the what but not the why or how. Students are also at risk of becoming dependent on AI for tasks like summarizing texts, solving problems, and creating outlines, which may have an effect on their own ability to perform these tasks independently [23, 24]. Educators must set expectations and guidelines for students that support ethical use of AI as a co-thinking agent and as a tool to expand modes of engagement with learning, not as a replacement for cognitive processing and deep learning.

Integrating StudyFetch into a Weekly Module For those new to AI integration, here's an example of how StudyFetch can be used in a course:

- *Course Module for a Given Topic*:
  - *Pre-Class*: The educator uploads key articles and slides to StudyFetch. The tool generates flashcards and a summary podcast for students' use.
  - *During Class*: Students complete a quick in-class quiz generated from StudyFetch. Educators review common errors in real time.
  - *Post-Class*: Students are instructed to ask StudyFetch for a brief explanation of any incorrect responses, then reflect on changes in their understanding in a shared discussion post. This approach takes minimal setup through the use of templates that are already embedded in the platform, but personalizes the learning pathway while giving educators real-time insights into student comprehension.
  - *Risk*: While many platforms use state-of-the-art model safeguards, there is an ongoing risk of bias and hallucinations. Many companies, like StudyFetch, could work to meticulously engineer AI search engines that are crafted to reduce bias and hallucinations; however, both remain a persistent challenge in AI because they arise from how large models learn and generate responses, not from correctable mistakes. Bias reflects the values, gaps, and distortions present in the training data, which mirror the real world and its inequities. Hallucination emerges from the need to synthesize language by aggregating partial, distributed knowledge under uncertainty. Together, they represent fundamental trade-offs in designing systems that are both expressive and useful. No amount of fine-tuning can fully eliminate them [25]. Educators should anticipate these issues and adequately prepare students to identify and address them as part of the learning experience.

5.3 Developing Clinical Judgment Through AI-Enhanced Simulation

Developing clinical judgment, the ability to assess, prioritize, and act decisively in complex patient situations, is one of the most critical and challenging goals in nursing education [26]. While helping students retain core knowledge is essential, they must also learn to apply that knowledge in dynamic clinical contexts. Traditionally, educators have used case studies, role-play, or limited-access simulation labs to move students toward this goal [27]. Today, AI-enhanced simulation tools offer new opportunities to expand, personalize, and deepen these experiences [5].

What distinguishes AI-supported simulation from traditional simulation is its adaptability and responsiveness [28]. Tools like Body Interact, Edocate, and Shadow Health create branching clinical scenarios that respond to student decisions in real time [29–31]. As a student selects interventions, delays in responding, or misses subtle cues, the scenario shifts, mimicking the evolving nature of real patient care. AI tracks not only outcomes but also how learners reach them, providing targeted feedback on reasoning, timeliness, and clinical priorities. These simulations aren't static; they are dynamic, formative spaces where students can build and refine clinical judgment safely and repeatedly.

AI makes simulation more accessible. In the past, high-quality simulation was often limited by cost, educator time, or lab space. AI-enhanced platforms can be used asynchronously, allowing students to engage on their own time while still receiving meaningful feedback. This provides individual experiences and expands opportunities for students who need more practice or are unable to participate fully in in-person sessions, and because scenarios can be personalized, learners receive practice that targets their growth areas rather than repeating content they've already mastered.

AI-generated simulation analytics offer a new layer of instructional insight. Educators can now review detailed performance data across clinical reasoning tasks, such as how long a student hesitated before intervening, whether they prioritized the correct symptoms, or how they navigated ethical decisions. AI-generated data can show that students may know content but struggle to apply that content in situations requiring early clinical judgment. These analytics help educators move beyond right-or-wrong scoring and instead see patterns of decision-making over time. Used well, this data supports real-time instructional adjustment and more tailored remediation.

Scenario A student repeatedly overlooks early signs of sepsis in a virtual patient simulation. The platform flags this pattern and recommends a targeted micro-scenario to reinforce critical thinking in time-sensitive conditions. At the same time, the educator sees similar patterns across the cohort and revises the next week's lecture to focus on recognizing subtle deterioration. This is the power of AI-enhanced simulation: personalized, data-informed, immediately actionable, and generalizable. (*For an AI tool to be generalizable, the tool must adapt to student needs, collect data, and rigorously evaluate students across diverse contexts*) [32].

AI simulation tools do not replace hands-on clinical learning, but can augment it and add dimensions of personalization. AI tools also free educators to spend more time mentoring and debriefing, focusing on reflective conversation rather than facilitating every aspect of the scenario. For students, AI-enabled simulations provide a low-stakes environment where it's safe to make mistakes, learn from them, and try again.

Scenario An experienced educator is tasked with writing a new case scenario for an upcoming lecture. Using an AI-powered simulation tool, the educator selects the target learning area or intended outcome. In response, the platform generates a recommended case scenario that includes presenting symptoms, relevant lab values, diagnostic distractors, and links to current evidence-based guidelines.

When intentionally aligned with course outcomes and paired with responsive instruction, AI-enhanced simulations can accelerate the development of clinical judgment, promote more equitable access to practice opportunities, and provide personalized feedback at scale [6, 28, 33]. Perhaps most importantly, they generate actionable data that helps educators see beyond performance scores to understand how students think, where they hesitate, and what supports are needed. These tools don't replace traditional instruction. They expand its reach, deepen impact, and provide the insights needed to help every learner grow.

5.4 Fostering Inquiry, Evidence Synthesis, and Research Literacy

Engaging in research can be daunting for nursing students, especially when they are still learning to critically appraise literature. Dense academic writing, unfamiliar terminology, and the sheer volume of available material often lead to cognitive overload [34, 35]. These challenges can hinder students' confidence and engagement with evidence-based practice before they have a chance to build foundational skills.

Artificial intelligence offers promising opportunities to scaffold the research process. When used effectively, AI tools can support students as they formulate questions, explore evidence, and synthesize findings. Developing the ability to ask meaningful, well-structured questions is a cornerstone of evidence-based practice [26, 36], and AI tools can play a valuable role in that development. For example, certain platforms can suggest keywords, map out conceptual relationships, or flag relevant studies that might otherwise go unnoticed.

By integrating AI into curriculum design, educators can lower barriers to scholarly inquiry while reinforcing essential competencies in research literacy, critical thinking, and synthesis [2, 5, 28]. The goal is not to replace human judgment but to enhance it. When used pedagogically, AI can help students navigate complex material without shortcutting rigor or critical engagement.

To achieve this, nursing programs must pair AI instruction with intentional education on its ethical and pedagogical use. Students need to understand not only how to use these tools, but also when and why to use them, preserving academic integrity and supporting their growth as thoughtful, curious, and evidence-informed professionals.

AI-supported research platforms such as Logically (formerly Afforai), Elicit, and ResearchRabbit offer students structured, interactive support for engaging with complex literature [37–39]. These tools allow users to upload portable document formats (PDFs) or pose research questions and receive citation-linked summaries that highlight key findings, themes, and methodological differences. Some platforms also help students organize ideas by generating synthesis scaffolds or suggested outlines. When integrated thoughtfully and paired with ethical guidance, these tools can lower access barriers to scholarly engagement, demystify the structure of academic writing, and support the development of higher-order reasoning and critical synthesis skills [2, 5, 40–42].

There is a scarcity of literature on *AI-supported research tools* and their impact on academic achievement; however, early studies point to AI supporting students' academic development [19, 43]. By reducing the cognitive load associated with initial article screening and synthesis, these platforms may lower the entry barrier to complex academic work, allowing students to spend more time analyzing content and making connections between sources [13, 22, 40]. While early evidence is emerging regarding AI-supported applications and student engagement with learning content, students who use AI-supported research tools engage more deeply with scholarly materials than they would through traditional means alone [3, 19]. An additional area ripe for investigation is whether students using these tools identify a broader range of relevant literature. While these hypotheses remain to be fully explored, the potential for AI to support more sustained and meaningful interaction with scholarly work remains a rapidly growing area of investigation.

Building on what is known about AI's potential to support learning, educators can consider designing research assignments that position AI not as a shortcut to answers, but as a catalyst for deeper inquiry. An example of one strategy is to have students engage with AI tools during the research or synthesis process, then reflect on how those tools influenced their thinking. By asking students to critically assess both the scholarly content and the AI's contribution, educators promote metacognition and digital literacy [44, 45]. This AI-supported research approach helps learners distinguish between information generation and understanding and builds the evaluative habits they will need to navigate AI-rich environments well beyond the classroom.

Example Assignment Using Research Supporting AI Software The following assignment encourages students to view AI as a collaborator, not a shortcut, while practicing evidence appraisal. Additionally, it reinforces critical appraisal while modeling AI as a thinking partner, not a shortcut [38].

Assignment Provide students with an assignment prompt such as, "Synthesize a response to a clinical question: What are the most effective nurse-led strategies for fall prevention in acute care?"

- *Step 1*: Use your selected software (such as Elicit or Logically) to upload and review at least three peer-reviewed articles written within the last 4 years. *Students should search using both Semantic Scholar and Google options within this platform.*
- *Step 2*: Generate a comparative summary using the platform's evidence synthesis tool.
- *Step 3*: Manually write a 250-word summary of findings, then a 150-word critique of how well Logically supported your synthesis. Highlight where you had to revise or add your own reasoning, focusing on the content highlighted by the Logically app within the source document.
- *Optional Step 4*: Conduct an academic library search and compare results. This step addresses the potential risk of over-reliance on an AI-driven database searches.

5.5 Enhancing Evidence-Based Practice Through AI-Assisted Literature Synthesis

In a senior-level nursing research course, educators aimed to bolster students' abilities in evidence-based practice by integrating AI tools into the curriculum. Recognizing the challenges students faced in navigating vast amounts of scholarly literature, the instructors introduced an assignment utilizing AI platforms such as Elicit and ResearchRabbit.

Assignment Structure
1. *Clinical Question Formulation*: Students began by developing a focused clinical question using the Population, Intervention, Comparison, Outcome (PICO) framework.
2. *Literature Search with AI Tools*: Using free versions of AI-supported tools like Elicit or Logically, students input their clinical questions to receive a curated list of relevant articles, complete with summaries and key findings. ResearchRabbit was employed to visualize connections between studies, helping students identify seminal works and research trends [37].
3. *Critical Appraisal*: Students selected a subset of articles for in-depth review.
4. *Synthesis and Reflection*: The final component involved uploading the results to Logically for support in synthesizing the findings into a coherent summary and reflecting on the AI tools' role in their research process.

Potential Outcomes

- *Structured Search Process*: AI tools guided students through an organized and efficient literature search, potentially reducing the time spent on irrelevant sources.
- *Enhanced Article Relevance*: The AI platforms' ability to suggest pertinent articles may have improved the quality of sources students engaged with.
- *Deeper Synthesis*: Visual mapping of research with an AI-tool, such as ResearchRabbit or AlphaSense, allowed students to understand the relationships between studies, fostering a nuanced synthesis of information.
- *Critical Thinking Development*: By evaluating the AI tools' suggestions and reflecting on their utility, students honed their critical appraisal skills and became more discerning consumers of information.

The above assignment examples are designed to illustrate how integrating AI tools into nursing education can enhance students' research capabilities, skills that are essential for effective evidence-based practice. The development of these assignments is based on the premise that early exposure to AI-supported research tools can better prepare students for scholarly inquiry. This is particularly critical in a healthcare landscape where such tools are becoming increasingly prevalent.

Integrating AI-supported research tools accomplishes more than streamlining the research process; it creates an opportunity to deepen students' engagement with scholarly work [3, 19]. When educators intentionally guide students to reflect on how AI contributes to their inquiry, they not only strengthen evidence-based practice but also nurture the habits of responsible digital scholarship [19, 28]. These tools can help students practice academic judgment, build confidence as emerging knowledge users and producers, and experience research as a space of exploration rather than intimidation. By embedding AI tools with care and transparency, educators can reframe inquiry as a collaborative process, one where human insight remains central, even in an era of machine assistance.

5.6 Promoting Reflection, Systems Thinking, and Professional Identity

In contemporary nursing education, fostering reflection, systems thinking, and a strong professional identity is critical to preparing practice-ready graduates. Reflection helps students make meaning from complex experiences and navigate uncertainty. Systems thinking enables students to recognize patterns, connections, and root causes within healthcare environments. Professional identity shapes how students see themselves as nurses; how they act, decide, and relate to others in ethical, patient-centered ways, yet these capacities do not develop automatically. Educators must intentionally design learning environments that nurture them, especially through dialogues, mentorship, and experiential learning. The following discussion explores how emerging AI tools can serve as partners in this developmental process.

Learning in nursing is not only cognitive; it is deeply relational, ethically situated, and reflective. Students are not just absorbing knowledge; students are becoming skilled professionals. This developmental process involves forming a sense of identity, understanding systems of care, grappling with moral complexity, and cultivating habits of reflection [46, 47], yet facilitating the development of professional identity through traditional educational methods, such as written journals or formal reflection, can be challenging. These assignments may feel performative or constrained, especially for learners still developing their professional voice. Some students may hesitate to express uncertainty or complexity in formal writing. What they need are low-stakes, dialogic opportunities to explore their thinking aloud, spaces where they can test ideas, reflect on values, and simulate the kind of reflective conversations that occur in clinical mentorship [48].

One promising avenue for supporting the development of reflection, systems thinking, and professional identity is the use of relational, or "co-thinking," AI tools [49]. Unlike static prompts or structured reflection templates, these tools simulate the dynamic back-and-forth of a mentoring conversation. Through interactive dialogue, students can articulate uncertainty, weigh ethical dimensions, and reflect in real time on how their thinking is taking shape. Whether guiding a student through a values conflict, a leadership dilemma, or a systems-level challenge, relational AI can provide a responsive, low-stakes environment that encourages exploration without judgment.

Relational AI tools work best when they are intentionally designed or carefully selected for reflective depth. For instance, a custom-built chatbot programmed to use Socratic questioning can walk students through an assignment by prompting them to consider alternatives, clarify reasoning, and trace cause and effect [42]. Developing a tool like this can be a relatively simple process when instructional goals are clearly defined. Even off-the-shelf tools, such as those found in the ChatGPT library or platforms like Boodlebox, can serve this purpose when introduced with guidance [43, 50, 51]. The key is not just the sophistication of the tool, but the way it is framed: as a partner in thinking, not a shortcut to completion.

An example of a custom-developed chatbot is Fishbone Coach, a chatbot designed to guide students through the process of completing a fishbone diagram in system-change courses [52]. Rather than giving students a template and expecting them to fill it in, the chatbot walks them through step-by-step reflection. Students engage with the bot iteratively, generating and revising ideas before producing a final fishbone diagram for educator feedback.

Similarly, ChatGPT and MagicSchool, for example, can be used, alongside clear student instructions, to generate reflection prompts, simulate ethical dilemmas, or support identity development through narrative inquiry [17, 50]. For example, in a leadership course, a student might ask ChatGPT to simulate a conversation with a resistant team member about implementing a new protocol. The tool would then help them explore tone, framing, and potential responses, then reflect on how their own communication style influences outcomes.

The use of an AI conversational agent that is designed, trained, and integrated to serve a unique purpose is especially valuable in courses emphasizing systems thinking, quality improvement, health equity, and leadership [42, 53]. These tools support learning that aligns with the American Association of Colleges of Nursing (AACN) Essentials, particularly domains related to ethical practice, professional formation, and person-centered care [1]. Student development activities via these tools can also reflect core principles from other competency frameworks, such as Quality and Safety Education for Nurses (QSEN's) emphasis on patient-centered care and safety, or the National League for Nursing (NLN's) focus on human flourishing, nursing judgment, and integrating technology in practice [54, 55]. With appropriate guidance and ethical parameters, chatbots can also reflect inclusive pedagogy, giving students private, low-stakes opportunities to explore their thinking, practice voice, and build confidence before sharing ideas more publicly [7, 56].

5.7 Use Case: Narrative Reflection and Identity Formation via AI Dialogue

Assignment Overview

In a professional formation or leadership course, students are asked to explore a moment in their clinical experience or coursework where they felt uncertain, challenged, or particularly affirmed in their identity as a future nurse. Using ChatGPT or a course-approved chatbot, students engage in a guided reflective dialogue, followed by a structured written response.

Instructions for Students

1. *Frame an Experience*: Identify a clinical or academic situation that prompted personal growth or ethical questioning. *Ensure de-identification of all information including location, names, dates or other identifying information.*

2. *Prompt the AI*: Ask the chatbot to simulate a reflective dialogue using a prompt such as:

   Act as a Socratic mentor, helping me reflect on a moment where I questioned my role as a nurse. Ask me open-ended questions to frame the circumstance, then help me explore my values and responses.

3. *Dialogue and Capture*: Engage with the chatbot for at least 10 exchanges. Save the transcript.

4. *Synthesize and Reflect*: Submit a one-page reflection addressing:
   - What insights emerged from the dialogue?
   - How did the chatbot's questions shape your thinking?
   - How does this moment inform your evolving professional identity?

5.8 Designing for Inclusion, Differentiation, and Flexible Learning Pathways

One of the most powerful promises of AI in nursing education lies in its potential to advance inclusion [7, 56]. Students arrive in classrooms with a wide range of lived experiences, abilities, responsibilities, learning needs, and neurodivergent profiles [57–59]. Many are balancing demanding roles outside of school, including caregiving responsibilities and part-time or full-time employment. Others speak English as an additional language or are navigating unspoken academic norms for the first time [60, 61]. Our educational systems do not always flex well to meet that diversity [59, 62]. And while AI cannot resolve structural inequities on its own, it can help us respond to learner differences with more nuance, creativity, and intention.

When integrated with intention, AI tools can enhance inclusive teaching practices without significantly increasing educator workload [7, 63]. Rather than replacing foundational pedagogy, these platforms offer scalable ways to honor learner variability. By supporting flexible pacing, generating multimodal content formats, and encouraging low-stakes practice, AI creates more access points for students to engage with complex material [7, 63]. These affordances align closely with the core principles of UDL, which emphasize multiple means of representation, expression, and engagement [64]. Through this lens, AI becomes not just a tool for efficiency but a partner in creating learning environments that are equitable by design.

Tools that personalize content delivery and adapt to different learning preferences, like MagicSchool and StudyFetch, allow students to transform dense course materials into flashcards, outlines, videos, or audio summaries [15, 17]. Interactive tools like Kahoot! and Curipod bring energy, visual engagement, and formative feedback into classroom settings [65, 66]. These platforms are especially valuable for students who may not thrive in traditional, text-heavy learning environments, offering alternative pathways for demonstrating understanding and participating in real time. AI-supported writing assistants can scaffold thinking and help students communicate complex ideas more effectively. For learners who might otherwise be overwhelmed by academic conventions, these tools reduce cognitive load and increase access without sacrificing academic rigor [63].

Educators can also apply AI tools in their own instructional design work. There are many chatbots available through ChatGPT, Boodlebox, and others that can assist with course and instructional design activities [50, 51]. For example, the Assignment Reviewer Pro chatbot supports inclusive course design by evaluating assignments for clarity, accessibility, and alignment with learning goals [67]. This allows educators to revise prompts or rubrics before students ever encounter them, proactively addressing barriers that might otherwise go unnoticed. In this model, the responsibility for inclusion shifts from student self-advocacy to thoughtful, equity-oriented design by the educator.

Another example is Jackson, a custom-developed chatbot created to provide feedback from the perspective of a neurodivergent, intersectional, Native nursing student [68]. Jackson engages with course materials, syllabi, assignments, and instructor feedback to help surface how content might be perceived by students from historically excluded or underserved backgrounds. While Jackson reflects the input of a single persona with reflections from one programmer's lived experience and does not claim to represent any group, the tool invites educators to consider how voice, tone, assumptions, and structural choices may affect learner experience. Used together, tools like Assignment Reviewer and Jackson encourage instructors to design with empathy, intersectionality, and inclusion at the center.

In addition to designing with inclusion in mind, educators can use analytics provided by many AI platforms to support equity during the course. Reviewing patterns of engagement or feedback can reveal gaps in tool usage or hidden obstacles that might disproportionately affect some students. Simple adjustments, such as offering multiple modalities for task completion or inviting feedback on AI-supported activities, can go a long way in helping students feel seen, supported, and respected.

Inclusive design is not a separate task from curriculum development [64]. It is the foundation of effective, learner-centered teaching and a model for patient-centered care. When AI tools are used to anticipate learner variability, affirm student agency, and reduce barriers to participation, educators are not just accommodating differences. They are building courses in which every student has the opportunity to thrive, and modeling mastery in nursing, a key motivational factor for all students [69].

Getting Started with AI in Your Course: A First Steps Guide Not sure where to begin? Start small:

1. *Pick one tool*—Try StudyFetch, MagicSchool, or ChatGPT based on your course needs.
2. *Start with one module*—Choose a high-volume or high-challenge week (e.g., med-surg, pharmacology). Add module learning content into your chosen tool (remember to avoid violating copyright laws).
3. *Set expectations*—Tell students what AI is (and isn't) meant to do. Frame AI as a support tool, a thinking partner, not a solution. Model ethical and critical use, and let your students experiment.
4. *Review, adapt, repeat*—Reflect on what worked, collect feedback, and scale gradually. Remember, the goal isn't perfection, it's progress. You don't need to master AI overnight. Just take one step forward and build from there.

5.9 Using AI-Supported Analytics to Inform Teaching and Learning

For years, nursing educators have had access to performance data. Simulation dashboards, Health Education Systems, Inc. (HESI) and Assessment Technologies Institute (ATI) reporting, and learning management system (LMS) analytics, for example, have all supported educators in identifying struggling students, spotting content gaps, and making targeted adjustments [31, 70]. These tools have supported instructional decision-making, curriculum mapping, and outcomes assessment. In many ways, this work has laid the foundation for reflective, data-informed teaching.

What makes AI-supported analytics different is not simply the volume of data they provide, but their ability to interpret it. AI systems go beyond recording right and wrong answers. They detect patterns across time and topic areas, uncover latent misconceptions, and recommend actionable next steps. Instead of presenting static dashboards, these platforms offer real-time, dynamic insight that supports just-in-time teaching, personalized remediation, and curriculum-level reflection [15, 17, 29].

For example, platforms like StudyFetch, MagicSchool, and Body Interact now offer educator dashboards that reveal where students hesitate, misapply knowledge, or demonstrate shallow understanding [15, 17, 29]. An instructor might see that learners are consistently struggling with medication titration in adaptive quizzes and delaying related interventions during simulation scenarios. These platforms can often expose class-level patterns as well, such as underperformance on application-level questions or declining engagement in later modules. Some AI-enhanced platforms take this a step further by suggesting instructional responses based on cross-sectional trends. If a student is struggling with fluid and electrolyte management, the system might recommend a related case study, a video walkthrough, or a simplified version of a prior concept. Instructors may also receive prompts to revisit a topic using a new modality, suggestions for peer review approaches, or to integrate a short, targeted review into the next class session. These small adjustments make instruction more responsive without requiring a complete redesign.

Another key advantage of AI analytics is the ability to track learning over time and across contexts [15, 17, 29]. Traditional tools offer snapshots, whereas AI offers storylines. For instance, if students repeatedly miss dosage calculation questions in multiple formats, the system might flag a pattern tied to content timing, prerequisite knowledge, or instructional alignment. This insight enables educators to address issues upstream in the course design, shifting from reactive to proactive teaching.

Case Study An educator in a pharmacology course used StudyFetch to review class-level analytics before a midterm module review. The dashboard showed a consistent dip in quiz performance following the introduction of cardiac medications, along with increased time-on-task and higher rates of incorrect first attempts. Rather than concluding that students simply needed more repetition, the instructor analyzed the underlying concepts and student feedback. They realized that while the content was clinically dense, the real barrier was cognitive overload; students were encountering new mechanisms of action, abbreviations, and calculations all at once, without time to process or connect the information to prior learning. In response, they redesigned the module by frontloading key vocabulary, embedding a guided pharmacokinetics activity, and introducing low-stakes quizzes that emphasized recognition before application. They also used a whiteboard flowchart activity in class to link drug types to clinical decision pathways. In the next term, student quiz accuracy and confidence ratings improved, and fewer questions appeared in the end-of-course review. The dashboard didn't offer a solution, but it helped prompt the right inquiry and guided the redesign with purpose.

The above use case illustrates the broader potential of AI analytics: not just showing us what is happening, but helping us ask why, and how we can intervene more meaningfully.

AI doesn't just help us see what students are doing. In some systems, it's beginning to show how they're thinking [15]. AI can analyze the complexity of student responses to determine whether their answers reflect recall, application, or analysis in Bloom's Revised Taxonomy [15, 20, 50]. It can detect whether clinical decisions are based on rule-following or emergent pattern recognition, aligning with frameworks like Tanner's Clinical Judgment Model or the National Council of State Boards of Nursing (NCSBN) Clinical Judgment Measurement Model [71, 72]. These insights help educators design interventions that support not only performance but cognitive development and professional formation.

To use these insights meaningfully, educators must stay actively engaged in interpretation. AI can detect trends, but it cannot assign contextual meaning. Educators must still ask: What does this tell me about how students are engaging? How does this connect to my course pacing, structure, or assessment design? Used reflectively, AI becomes a co-instructor, not just a measurement tool.

AI's ability to surface detailed insights also raises ethical responsibilities. The more granular our visibility becomes, the greater our obligation to use that information transparently and equitably. Students should understand what data is collected, how it will be used, and who has access [7]. Informed consent, data minimization, and clear communication must be embedded from the outset. To support ethical implementation, Kaliisa, Jivet, and Prinsloo [73] offer a four-dimensional framework for evaluating learning analytics systems. Their model encourages institutions to align data use with pedagogical purpose, involve stakeholders in tool selection, and embed ethical principles throughout the analytics lifecycle. As more educators adopt AI-enhanced platforms, this kind of scaffolding becomes essential to ensure both instructional and ethical soundness [7, 56, 70]. When students see analytics as a tool for learning, rather than surveillance, trust grows, and so does engagement.

Used thoughtfully, AI analytics do not replace educator expertise; they extend it. These tools help us move beyond identifying who is struggling to understanding why, how, and when those struggles emerge. They allow us to teach more proactively, support more responsively, and design more intentionally, not through guesswork, but through evidence, delivered when it matters most.

5.10 Use Case: Analytics for Just-in-Time Teaching (JiTT)

What to Do
Before each class, review the dashboard from your adaptive tool (e.g., StudyFetch, MagicSchool, Body Interact) to identify:

- Common misconceptions
- Most-missed quiz questions
- Low-engagement content areas

How to Do It

Use this to revise *only* 10–15 minutes of your planned lecture and address the confusion head-on with a mini-case, poll, or demo. Ask the class for feedback and refine or continue with your lecture. Clearing up difficult points for students early in learning lessens cognitive load and helps students be more prepared to learn. This strategy makes teaching adaptive without being time-intensive. Bonus: Students see that their effort shapes class time, increasing engagement.

5.11 Use Case: Add a "Data-Informed Reflection" Assignment

What to Do

Ask students to review their analytics dashboard (from StudyFetch or Body Interact) and submit:

- A summary of 1–2 learning strengths
- A plan for addressing 1 learning gap
- A critique of the dashboard's usefulness

Why It Works

This strategy builds metacognition and prepares students to interpret data, crucial for both lifelong learning and real-world clinical practice.

5.12 Aligning AI Integration with Curriculum and Program Outcomes

Effective AI integration begins with clarity of purpose. Educators do not need to master every tool or trend. Instead, they must anchor instructional decisions in the learning outcomes they've already committed to, whether course objectives, program competencies, clinical performance expectations, the AACN Essentials, or frameworks such as QSEN and the NLN Core Competencies [1, 54, 55]. These outcomes provide the framework. AI becomes a set of tools that help realize those intentions more effectively, equitably, and responsively.

Using a backward design approach, educators can begin by asking what students should be able to know, do, and demonstrate [74]. With those outcomes in mind, educators can select AI tools that reinforce skill development, provide timely feedback, or make invisible thinking processes visible. For example, if a course outcome emphasizes interprofessional communication, educators might incorporate ChatGPT to simulate difficult conversations [50]. If a program outcome calls for the application of quality improvement methods, the Fishbone Coach chatbot could help guide students through root cause analysis as part of a systems-based intervention project [52].

AI-supported platforms also offer new ways to monitor and reinforce alignment across multiple levels:

- *Lesson and module level*: AI tools like MagicSchool and Curipod can generate exit tickets, quizzes, or discussion prompts that map directly to module objectives. Educators can use these to assess immediate understanding and adjust instruction accordingly.
- *Course level*: Adaptive simulations or interactive cases can serve as formative or summative assessments aligned with course learning outcomes, such as demonstrating clinical judgment, ethical reasoning, or care prioritization. Dashboards from platforms like Edocate or Body Interact offer real-time insights into student engagement and performance.
- *Program level*: AI-generated analytics can support curriculum committees and program directors by identifying patterns in student learning across courses. These trends may signal areas for redesign, faculty development, or curricular scaffolding. For instance, if multiple cohorts underperform on pharmacological calculations in simulation, educators might revise instruction in both pathophysiology and clinical lab courses.

Mapping AI tool learning experiences to existing competency frameworks strengthens this alignment. For example:

- A tool that supports adaptive learning content: Map the learning content and learning goals as appropriate to AACN Essentials Domain 1 (Knowledge for Nursing Practice), QSEN's Knowledge and Safety dimensions, or NLN Competency 1: Human Flourishing.
- An AI-supported simulation platform learning goals: Map the content and goals as appropriate to support Domain 6 (Interprofessional Partnerships) and QSEN's Teamwork and Collaboration, while also aligning with NLN Competency 4: Person-Centered Care.
- AI writing assistants or inquiry bots: Map assignments supporting reflection, identity formation, and lifelong learning, consistent with AACN Domains 5, 9, and 10, QSEN's Patient-Centered Care, and NLN Competency 8: Professionalism and Leadership.

When used thoughtfully, AI tools can create a thread of coherence across the curriculum, not by standardizing experiences, but by creating consistent access to feedback, reinforcement, and reflection. This enhances both student learning and curriculum integrity.

Alignment with AI tools does not mean rigidity. Educators may begin with one aligned AI-enhanced assignment, observe its effect, and iterate over time. As instructors become more confident, they can scale integration across courses and levels, gradually building a responsive, AI-supported learning ecosystem. The evolving landscape of AI in education necessitates that nurse educators engage in continuous professional development to effectively integrate these technologies. Faculty development programs focusing on digital literacy, ethical considerations, and pedagogical strategies are essential. Such initiatives empower educators to critically assess AI tools, align them with curricular goals, and model responsible use for students [28].

Ultimately, alignment is about ensuring that AI serves the curriculum, and not the reverse. When used with intention and anchored to clear learning outcomes, AI can become a powerful partner in designing learning that prepares students not only for today's clinical demands but for the emerging realities of tomorrow's practice.

5.13 Leading with Purpose in the AI Era

The integration of artificial intelligence into nursing education is a pressing opportunity. As educators, we are navigating a landscape where both clinical practice and learner expectations are evolving rapidly. AI offers powerful tools to meet this moment, but only when deployed with intentionality, ethics, humility, and a clear connection to our pedagogical values [56].

Throughout this chapter, we have explored how AI can support knowledge acquisition, clinical judgment, inquiry, reflection, inclusion, and alignment with curricular outcomes. These are not isolated tasks. They form the interconnected work of preparing nurses who think critically, act ethically, and adapt skillfully in a healthcare system increasingly shaped by digital tools.

Importantly, integrating AI does not require mastery of every platform. It requires curiosity. As educators, we can model the mindset we hope to cultivate in our students: one of experimentation, iterative growth, and reflective adaptation [43]. Whether starting with a single lesson, a challenging concept, or a course already under revision, the goal is not to overhaul everything at once, but to begin, observe, and build thoughtfully from what works.

AI should never replace the human elements of teaching: relationships, mentorship, or the ability to recognize and nurture potential. Instead, it can extend our reach, sharpen our insight, and enable more responsive, equitable, and inclusive learning. As AI becomes more embedded in academic life, educators are increasingly responsible for guiding ethical classroom use, selecting tools that align with core values, and addressing concerns around data privacy, algorithmic bias, and accessibility [7, 56, 75]. These responsibilities are not tangential; they are central to shaping a future in which innovation strengthens, rather than compromises, the heart of nursing education.

More than integrators, nurse educators are also potential co-designers. By partnering with developers, educators can help shape AI systems that reflect nursing pedagogy, clinical nuance, and the values of justice, equity, and inclusion. Educators are uniquely positioned to offer input on tool functionality, learner needs, and competency alignment, ensuring that emerging technologies are built with, rather than imposed upon, the profession.

Table 5.1 Practical AI tools for nursing education: applications and considerations

Tool	Primary function	Educational application	Considerations
StudyFetch	Adaptive learning and study aid	Personalized quizzes and flashcards for content reinforcement	Ensure content accuracy and alignment with course objectives
MagicSchool AI	Content generation and lesson planning	Assists in creating lesson plans and formative assessments	Review AI-generated content for pedagogical appropriateness
Body Interact	Virtual patient simulations	Enhances clinical decision-making through interactive scenarios	Supplement with debriefing sessions to reinforce learning
ChatGPT	Conversational AI for tutoring and reflection	Facilitates student engagement in ethical dilemmas and Q&A, and offers Study Mode	Monitor for accuracy and encourage critical evaluation of responses
Fishbone Coach	Guided root cause analysis tool	Supports systems thinking in quality improvement projects	Provide guidance on interpreting AI suggestions within context

Note: Ensure that the use of these tools complies with your institutional policies and ethical standards

The AI era is not about replacing educators, it is about empowering them. Through careful design, critical reflection, and bold experimentation, we can create learning environments that rise to this moment and prepare nurses who will do the same. The intent of this chapter was to help educators plan and model the ethical approaches to teaching and learning for future professionals.

The following chart illustrates the various functions and applications of AI tools that can be used to augment teaching and learning. The authors recognize some educators may believe that the easy availability of AI generated content can lead to or facilitate plagiarism and decrease critical thinking and problem-solving skills. Yes, overreliance on AI tools could potentially lead to the graduation of students who over-rely on artificial intelligence and underutilize critical thinking skills (Table 5.1).

References

1. AACN. The essentials [Internet]. 2025 [cited 2025 Feb 14]. Available from: https://www.aacnnursing.org/essentials.
2. Nguyen T. ChatGPT in medical education: a precursor for automation bias? JMIR Med Educ [Internet]. 2024;10:e50174. Available from: https://doi.org/10.2196/50174.
3. Bhatia A, Bhatia P, Sood D. Leveraging AI to transform online higher education: focusing on personalized learning, assessment, and student engagement. Int J Manag Humanit [Internet]. 2024 [cited 2025 May 9];11(1):1–6. Available from: https://www.ijmh.org/portfolio-item/A175311010924/.
4. Vorsah RE, Oppong F. Leveraging AI to enhance active learning strategies in science classrooms: implications for teacher professional development. World J Adv Res Rev [Internet].

2024 [cited 2025 Feb 27];24(2):1355–70. Available from: https://wjarr.com/content/leveraging-ai-enhance-active-learning-strategies-science-classrooms-implications-teacher.

5. Villegas-Ch W, Govea J, Gutierrez R, Mera-Navarrete A. Improving interaction and assessment in a hybrid educational environment: an integrated approach in Microsoft teams with the use of AI techniques. IEEE Access. 2024;12:93723–38.

6. Liu K, Zhang W, Li W, Wang T, Zheng Y. Effectiveness of virtual reality in nursing education: a systematic review and meta-analysis. BMC Med Educ [Internet]. 2023 [cited 2025 Aug 3];23(1):710. Available from: https://bmcmededuc.biomedcentral.com/articles/10.1186/s12909-023-04662-x.

7. Nikolopoulou K. Generative artificial intelligence in higher education: exploring ways of harnessing pedagogical practices with the assistance of ChatGPT. Int J Chang Educ [Internet]. 2024 [cited 2025 May 10];1(2):103–11. Available from: https://ojs.bonviewpress.com/index.php/IJCE/article/view/2489.

8. McHugh D, Yanik AJ, Mancini MR. An innovative pharmacology curriculum for medical students: promoting higher order cognition, learner-centered coaching, and constructive feedback through a social pedagogy framework. BMC Med Educ [Internet]. 2021 [cited 2025 May 9];21(1):90. Available from: https://bmcmededuc.biomedcentral.com/articles/10.1186/s12909-021-02516-y.

9. Neu T, Johnson AM. Journey of a drug: teaching pharmacokinetics and pharmacodynamics. Teach Learn Nurs [Internet]. 2024 [cited 2025 May 9];19(3):e580–3. Available from: https://linkinghub.elsevier.com/retrieve/pii/S155730872400091X.

10. Liu K, Lahoz EA. Impact of learning styles on students' retention of information. Int J Educ Humanit [Internet]. 2024 [cited 2025 May 9];17(1):207–12. Available from: https://drpress.org/ojs/index.php/ijeh/article/view/27006.

11. Gassas R. Sources of the knowledge-practice gap in nursing: Lessons from an integrative review. Nurse Educ Today [Internet]. 2021 [cited 2025 May 9];106:105095. Available from: https://linkinghub.elsevier.com/retrieve/pii/S026069172100352X.

12. Berdida DJE, Lopez V, Grande RAN. Nursing students' perceived stress, social support, self-efficacy, resilience, mindfulness and psychological well-being: a structural equation model. Int J Ment Health Nurs [Internet]. 2023 [cited 2025 May 9];32(5):1390–404. Available from: https://onlinelibrary.wiley.com/doi/abs/10.1111/inm.13179.

13. Khotimah K, Rusijono, Mariono A. Enhancing metacognitive and creativity skills through AI-driven meta-learning strategies. Int J Interact Mob Technol IJIM [Internet]. 2024 [cited 2025 Feb 27];18(05):18–31. Available from: https://online-journals.org/index.php/i-jim/article/view/47705.

14. Yue S. The evolution of pedagogical theory: from traditional to modern approaches and their impact on student engagement and success. J Educ Educ Res [Internet]. 2024 [cited 2025 Feb 27];7(3):226–30. Available from: https://drpress.org/ojs/index.php/jeer/article/view/18761.

15. Study Fetch. The top AI learning platform [Internet]. 2025 [cited 2025 Apr 25]. Available from: https://www.studyfetch.com/.

16. Quizlet. Study tools & learning resources for students and teachers [Internet]. 2025 [cited 2025 May 1]. Available from: https://quizlet.com/.

17. MagicSchool. AI for educators [Internet]. 2025 [cited 2025 Apr 25]. Available from: https://www.magicschool.ai/.

18. McMurtie B. The future is hybrid: colleges begin to reimagine learning in an AI world. The Chronicle of Higher Education; 2024.

19. Vieriu AM, Petrea G. The impact of artificial intelligence (AI) on students' academic development. Educ Sci [Internet]. 2025 [cited 2025 May 9];15(3):343. Available from: https://www.mdpi.com/2227-7102/15/3/343.

20. Krathwohl DR. A revision of bloom's taxonomy: an overview. Theory Pract [Internet]. 2002 [cited 2025 Aug 3];41(4):212–8. Available from: https://www.tandfonline.com/doi/full/10.1207/s15430421tip4104_2.

21. Marks B, Sisirak J. Nurses with disability: transforming healthcare for all. OJIN Online J Issues Nurs [Internet]. 2022 [cited 2025 Aug 3];27(3). Available from: https://ojin.nursingworld.org/table-of-contents/volume-27-2022/number-3-september-2022/nurses-with-disability/.

22. Mihmas Mesfer Aldawsari M, Rashed Ibrahim Almohish N. Threats and opportunities of students' use of AI-integrated technology (ChatGPT) in online higher education: Saudi Arabian educational technologists' perspectives. Int Rev Res Open Distrib Learn [Internet]. 2024 [cited 2025 May 9];25(3):19–36. Available from: https://www.irrodl.org/index.php/irrodl/article/view/7642.

23. Hernandez HE, Manalese RP, Dianelo RFB, Yambao JA, Gamboa AB, Feliciano LD, et al. Dependency on meta AI Chatbot in messenger among STEM and non-STEM students in higher education. Int J Comput Sci. 2025;9:3674–90.

24. Elbadiansyah, Sain ZH, Shehu Lawal U, Chansa Thelma C, Luqman Aziz A. Exploring the role of artificial intelligence in enhancing student motivation and cognitive development in higher education. TechComp Innov J Comput Sci Technol [Internet]. 2024 [cited 2025 Aug 3];1(2):59–67. Available from: https://mabadiiqtishada.org/index.php/TechCompInnovations/article/view/47.

25. Karpowicz MP. On the fundamental impossibility of hallucination control in large language models [Internet]. arXiv. 2025 [cited 2025 Aug 3]. Available from: http://arxiv.org/abs/2506.06382.

26. AACN. AACN essentials [Internet]. 2021 [cited 2025 Jan 2]. Available from: https://www.aacnnursing.org/essentials.

27. Weeks K, Herron E, Buchanan H. Aligning simulation-based education with didactic learning in prelicensure baccalaureate nursing education. Nurse Educ [Internet]. 2024 [cited 2025 Aug 3];49(3):125–9. Available from: https://journals.lww.com/10.1097/NNE.0000000000001554.

28. Labrague LJ, Al Sabei S, Al Yahyaei A. Artificial intelligence in nursing education: a review of AI-based teaching pedagogies. Teach Learn Nurs [Internet]. 2025 [cited 2025 May 9]:S1557308725000307. Available from: https://linkinghub.elsevier.com/retrieve/pii/S1557308725000307.

29. Nursing Education [Internet]. Body interact. Available from: https://bodyinteract.com/nursing-us/.

30. Edocate VPS [Internet]. [cited 2025 May 9]. Edocate. Available from: https://www.edocate.com/edocate-vps/.

31. Elsevier. www.elsevier.com. 2025 [cited 2025 May 1]. Shadow health digital standardized patients. Available from: https://www.elsevier.com/products/shadow-health/patients.

32. García FP, Cánovas Ó, Clemente FJG. Exploring AI techniques for generalizable teaching practice identification. IEEE Access [Internet]. 2024 [cited 2025 Aug 3];12:134702–13. Available from: https://ieeexplore.ieee.org/document/10670386/.

33. Sharon C, Green G. Life-threatening clinical simulations for nursing students: promoting critical thinking and satisfaction. J Nurs Educ [Internet]. 2024 [cited 2025 Aug 3];63(9):595–603. Available from: https://journals.healio.com/doi/10.3928/01484834-20240507-03.

34. Daniel B. Common challenges postgraduate students and early-career academics face when engaging with the scholarly literature. Electron J Bus Res Methods [Internet]. 2022 [cited 2025 Aug 3];20(3):142–52. Available from: https://academic-publishing.org/index.php/ejbrm/article/view/2503.

35. Zhang M, Doi L, Awua J, Asare H, Stenhouse R. Challenges and possible solutions for accessing scholarly literature among medical and nursing professionals and students in low-and-middle income countries: a systematic review. Nurse Educ Today [Internet]. 2023 [cited 2025 Aug 3];123:105737. Available from: https://linkinghub.elsevier.com/retrieve/pii/S026069172300031X.

36. Abu-Baker NN, AbuAlrub S, Obeidat RF, Assmairan K. Evidence-based practice beliefs and implementations: a cross-sectional study among undergraduate nursing students. BMC Nurs [Internet]. 2021 [cited 2025 Aug 3];20(1):13. Available from: https://bmcnurs.biomedcentral.com/articles/10.1186/s12912-020-00522-x.

37. Reimagine Research [Internet]. [cited 2025 May 9]. ResearchRabbit. Available from: https://www.researchrabbit.ai/.

38. Logically.app (formerly Afforai) | Everything you need to write a kick-ass paper, in one place. [Internet]. [cited 2025 Aug 2]. Available from: https://afforai.com/.

39. About Elicit [Internet]. [cited 2025 May 9]. Elicit. Available from: https://support.elicit.com/en/categories/146369-about-elicit.

40. AbuSahyon ASE, Alzyoud A, Alshorman O, Al-Absi B. AI-driven technology and Chatbots as tools for enhancing English language learning in the context of second language acquisition: a review study. Int J Membr Sci Technol [Internet]. 2023 [cited 2025 Aug 3];10(1):1209–23. Available from: https://cosmosscholars.com/phms/index.php/ijmst/article/view/2829.

41. Kashkin V, Androsik Y. Automated assessment of leadership style and professional values of a top-manager and its compliance with SDGS. J Lifestyle SDGs Rev [Internet]. 2024 [cited 2025 May 10];5(2):e03336. Available from: https://sdgsreview.org/LifestyleJournal/article/view/3336.

42. Krauter J. Bridging the Uncanny Valley: improving AI Chatbots for effective leadership mentoring. Open J Leadersh [Internet]. 2024 [cited 2025 May 10];13(03):342–84. Available from: https://www.scirp.org/journal/doi.aspx?doi=10.4236/ojl.2024.133021.

43. Wang J, Fan W. The effect of ChatGPT on students' learning performance, learning perception, and higher-order thinking: insights from a meta-analysis. Humanit Soc Sci Commun [Internet]. 2025 [cited 2025 May 10];12(1):621. Available from: https://www.nature.com/articles/s41599-025-04787-y.

44. Fox E, Riconscente M. Metacognition and self-regulation in James, Piaget, and Vygotsky. Educ Psychol Rev [Internet]. 2008 [cited 2025 Aug 3];20(4):373–89. Available from: http://link.springer.com/10.1007/s10648-008-9079-2.

45. Naamati-Schneider L. Enhancing AI competence in health management: students' experiences with ChatGPT as a learning tool. BMC Med Educ [Internet]. 2024 [cited 2025 May 10];24(1):598. Available from: https://bmcmededuc.biomedcentral.com/articles/10.1186/s12909-024-05595-9.

46. Batterbee R, Bradshaw J, Frost A, Hunt S. The use of a cognitive behavioural model of reflection to facilitate transformative learning in undergraduate nursing education. The quantitative results of a mixed methods study. Nurse Educ Pract [Internet]. 2025 [cited 2025 Aug 3];87:104444. Available from: https://linkinghub.elsevier.com/retrieve/pii/S1471595325002008.

47. Page S, Murray S, Gill SK, Johnston S. Connection pedagogy: a relational approach to nursing education. Int J Hum Caring [Internet]. 2025 [cited 2025 Aug 3];29(2):110–6. Available from: http://connect.springerpub.com/lookup/doi/10.20467/IJHC-2023-0033.

48. Boyd VA, Woods NN, Kumagai AK, Kawamura AA, Orsino A, Ng SL. Examining the impact of dialogic learning on critically reflective practice. Acad Med [Internet]. 2022 [cited 2025 Aug 3];97(11S):S71–9. Available from: https://journals.lww.com/10.1097/ACM.0000000000004916.

49. Bearman M, Ajjawi R. Learning to work with the black box: pedagogy for a world with artificial intelligence. Br J Educ Technol [Internet]. 2023 [cited 2025 May 10];54(5):1160–73. Available from: https://bera-journals.onlinelibrary.wiley.com/doi/10.1111/bjet.13337.

50. Introducing ChatGPT [Internet]. [cited 2025 May 10]. OpenAI. Available from: https://openai.com/index/chatgpt/.

51. About Us [Internet]. [cited 2025 May 10]. BoodleBox. Available from: https://boodlebox.ai/about/.

52. La Rosa D. Fishbone Coach. 2025 [cited 2025 May 10]. Fishbone Coach. Available from: https://chatgpt.com/g/g-67d372a92bc4819191b03bf23257001a-fishbone-coach.

53. The Learning Health System Series, National Academy of Medicine. Generative artificial intelligence in health and medicine: opportunities and responsibilities for transformative innovation [Internet]. Maddox T, Babski D, Embi P, Gerhart J, Goldsack J, Parikh R, et al., editors. Washington, DC: National Academies Press; 2025 [cited 2025 May 9]. Available from: https://nap.nationalacademies.org/catalog/28907.

54. QSEN Institute Competencies [Internet]. [cited 2025 May 10]. QSEN. Available from: https://www.qsen.org/competencies-pre-licensure-ksas.

55. Default [Internet]. [cited 2025 Aug 3]. Competencies for graduates of nursing programs. Available from: https://www.nln.org/education/nursing-education-competencies/competencies-for-graduates-of-nursing-programs.

56. Srinivasan M, Venugopal A, Venkatesan L, Kumar R. Navigating the pedagogical landscape: exploring the implications of AI and Chatbots in nursing education. JMIR Nurs [Internet]. 2024 [cited 2025 May 10];7:e52105. Available from: https://nursing.jmir.org/2024/1/e52105.

57. Major R, Jackson C, Wareham J, Pidcock J. Supporting neurodivergent nursing students in their practice placements. Nurs Stand [Internet]. 2024 [cited 2025 Aug 3];39(7):57–65. Available from: https://journals.rcni.com/doi/10.7748/ns.2024.e12262.

58. Jackson BL, Cameron VK, Hodgens TM, Jamal-Eddine SA, Kunte V, Marsala-Cervasio K, et al. Disability and accommodation use in US Bachelor of Science in Nursing Programs. JAMA Netw Open [Internet]. 2025 [cited 2025 Aug 3];8(2):e2461038. Available from: https://jamanetwork.com/journals/jamanetworkopen/fullarticle/2830457.

59. Zappas M, Walton-Moss B, Sanchez C, Hildebrand JA, Kirkland T. The decolonization of nursing education. J Nurse Pract [Internet]. 2021 [cited 2025 Aug 3];17(2):225–9. Available from: https://linkinghub.elsevier.com/retrieve/pii/S1555415520306061.

60. Wilcox MM, Pietrantonio KR, Farra A, Franks DN, Garriott PO, Burish EC. Stalling at the starting line: first-generation college students' debt, economic stressors, and delayed life milestones in professional psychology. Train Educ Prof Psychol [Internet]. 2022 [cited 2025 Aug 3];16(4):315–24. Available from: https://doi.apa.org/doi/10.1037/tep0000385.

61. Osakwe ZT, Obioha CU, Minuti A, Atairu M, Osborne JC. Barriers and facilitators to success in undergraduate nursing education among minority students: a systematic review. Nurse Educ [Internet]. 2022 [cited 2025 Aug 3];47(2):E18–23. Available from: https://journals.lww.com/10.1097/NNE.0000000000001154.

62. Sumpter D, Blodgett N, Beard K, Howard V. Transforming nursing education in response to the future of nursing 2020–2030 report. Nurs Outlook [Internet]. 2022 [cited 2025 May 1];70(6):S20–31. Available from: https://linkinghub.elsevier.com/retrieve/pii/S0029655422000197.

63. Lee SS, Moore RL. Harnessing generative AI (GenAI) for automated feedback in higher education: a systematic review. Online Learn [Internet]. 2024 [cited 2025 May 10];28(3). Available from: https://olj.onlinelearningconsortium.org/index.php/olj/article/view/4593.

64. Hills M, Overend A, Hildebrandt S. Faculty perspectives on UDL: exploring bridges and barriers for broader adoption in higher education. Can J Scholarsh Teach Learn [Internet]. 2022 [cited 2025 Aug 3];13(1). Available from: https://ojs.lib.uwo.ca/index.php/cjsotl_rcacea/article/view/13588.

65. Curipod. Curipod. 2025 [cited 2025 May 1]. Feel the buzz of 100% participation. Available from: https://curipod.com/.

66. Kahoot! Learning games: make learning awesome! [Internet]. 2025 [cited 2025 May 1]. Available from: https://kahoot.com/.

67. La Rosa D. Assignment Reviewer Pro. 2025 [cited 2025 May 10]. Assignment Reviewer Pro. Available from: https://chatgpt.com/g/g-67511f37f9bc8191968aded763d0ad68-assignment-reviewer-pro.

68. Jackson [Internet]. 2025 [cited 2025 May 10]. Jackson. Available from: https://chatgpt.com/g/g-6806791efd2c81919c80771b117286be-jackson.

69. Erlam GD. Are they watching: pedagogical influence of role modeling on student competence, confidence, and clinical reasoning. Open J Nurs [Internet]. 2022 [cited 2025 Aug 3];12(06):411–27. Available from: https://www.scirp.org/journal/doi.aspx?doi=10.4236/ojn.2022.126028.

70. Main [Internet]. [cited 2025 Aug 3]. Educator support & resources | ATI. Available from: https://www.atitesting.com/educator/suport-and-resources.

71. NCLEX [Internet]. [cited 2025 Aug 3]. Clinical judgment measurement model. Available from: https://nclex.com/clinical-judgment-measurement-model.page.

72. Tanner CA. Thinking like a nurse: a research-based model of clinical judgment in nursing. J Nurs Educ [Internet]. 2006 [cited 2025 Aug 3];45(6):204–11. Available from: https://journals.healio.com/doi/10.3928/01484834-20060601-04.

73. Kaliisa R, Jivet I, Prinsloo P. A checklist to guide the planning, designing, implementation, and evaluation of learning analytics dashboards. Int J Educ Technol High Educ [Internet]. 2023 [cited 2025 May 10];20(1):28. Available from: https://educationaltechnologyjournal.springeropen.com/articles/10.1186/s41239-023-00394-6.

74. Rinaldi K, Messer M, Hanson A, Chan J. Utilization of backward design in health professional education: a rapid review. J Prof Nurs [Internet]. 2025 [cited 2025 Aug 3];58:31–8. Available from: https://linkinghub.elsevier.com/retrieve/pii/S8755722325000237.

75. El Arab RA, Al Moosa OA, Abuadas FH, Somerville J. The role of AI in nursing education and practice: umbrella review. J Med Internet Res [Internet]. 2025 [cited 2025 Apr 5];27:e69881. Available from: https://www.jmir.org/2025/1/e69881.

A.I.'s Impact on Nursing Practice and Care

6

Rachel Rae Walker, Seyyedehmahdiyeh Khastar, Francis Kuehnle, and Miaomiao Shen

6.1 Introduction

Nursing is a uniquely human service for human beings who are served by, not controlled by, human technological creations. Maintaining the influence of technological competency as caring in nursing within the complex world of nursing is critical to sustaining a mutually rewarding engagement between the nurse and the one nursed.

—Rozzano C. Locsin & Marguerite Purnell, authors of "Advancing the Theory of Technological Competency as Caring in Nursing: The Universal Technological Domain" [1] p. 53

AI needs to be brought back down to earth. It has been elevated to a superhuman level that leads us to believe it is both inevitable and beyond our control. When AI research, development and deployment is rooted in people and communities from the start, we can get in front of these harms and create a future that values equity and humanity.

—Timnit Gebru, Founder of the Distributed A.I. Research Institute [Press Release]

R. R. Walker (✉) · S. Khastar · M. Shen
Elaine Marieb College of Nursing, University of Massachusetts Amherst, Amherst, MA, USA
e-mail: r.walker@umass.edu; skhastar@umass.edu; miaomiaoshen@umass.edu

F. Kuehnle
Nursing, The Providence Center, Providence, RI, USA
e-mail: FKuehnle@CareNE.org

© The Author(s), under exclusive license to Springer Nature Switzerland AG 2026
D. W. La Rosa et al. (eds.), *Nursing Education in the AI Era*,
https://doi.org/10.1007/978-3-032-12402-9_6

Chapter Learning Objectives

(a) Describe how A.I. in clinical care impacts nurses and nursing futures.
(b) Explore current and predicted roles for A.I. in clinical workflows and decision-making.
(c) Analyze cases of A.I. use in predictive analytics, diagnostics, and team collaboration.
(d) Address patient care quality, safety, and consent in the context of A.I.

Artificial intelligence (A.I.) is increasingly impacting nursing and health care. Whether nurses embrace A.I. or not, our care and clinical environments are increasingly shaped by these technologies. Nurses who seek to exercise sound clinical judgment in the context of A.I. should understand the advantages and limitations of these applications [1]. To practice ethically, nurses must also engage with established harms of A.I. to patients and the planet [2]. This chapter explores A.I.'s impacts on nurses' and patients' safety and well-being, collaboration and clinical decision-making, and nursing practice.

6.2 Defining Our Terms

Defining A.I.'s role in nursing and health care can be confusing, in part, because "A.I." in the wild is a marketing term, rather than a coherent set of technologies [3]. A.I. is an intentionally ambiguous concept whose definition continues to evolve in relation to power [4]. "A.I." often refers to computers performing tasks that resemble those which might otherwise require human intelligence [5]. The term is frequently used synonymously with terms like "machine learning," a field of inquiry in mathematics and engineering sciences whose roots date back to the 1950s. A.I. technologies encompass multiple sub-fields, methodologies, and technical innovations such as computer vision, neural networks, deep learning, generative A.I., natural language processing, and robotics. Agentic A.I. is an emerging application. A.I. agents are chatbots that can engage patients to provide some types of structured assessment, patient education, motivational interviewing, and referrals. Unlike generative A.I. applications like ChatGPT that require users to provide specific prompts, A.I. agents are designed to function autonomously.

On the Importance of Standpoint A standpoint is a position from which an issue is viewed, presented, and judged. *All* discussions of A.I. come from one or more standpoints. The function, application, and impacts of A.I. technologies are a product of power and decision-making, including who is included in decisions about A.I., who benefits from this arrangement, and who is harmed [6]. Therefore when discussing A.I., it is important to understand the lens through which the source approaches the discussion. As authors, we've included statements summarizing our respective positionalities vis-à-vis this topic at the end of a chapter. Our discussion is grounded in the following concepts, which serve as cross-cutting themes throughout the rest of this chapter: health justice, consent, sustainability, invisible labor, and digital defense. Case examples feature nursing considerations related to each of these concepts.

Health Justice Health justice is defined as an "equitable redistribution of power and resources such that people with the greatest need are prioritized, and where the processes of knowledge production around need, restructuring, and redistribution are grounded in the experiences of populations most impacted by health inequities" [7]. In the context of A.I., health justice is a paradigm that examines the socio-technical systems, structures, institutions, and power dynamics that create and perpetuate health inequities. Right now power over A.I.'s infrastructure is concentrated in the hands of industry executives and technologists disproportionately located in the Global North, with many headquartered in the A.I. hub of Silicon Valley. The Silicon Valley Pain Index measures wealth inequality in the region. The most recent index (released on July 14, 2025) revealed 0.1% of households hold 71% of the total wealth of the region, and just 0.01% of the population possess a whopping 15%. This growing wealth gap reflects the extractive nature of Silicon Valley, whose top executives inhabit a wholly different socio-economic sphere than the majority of populations their products surveil and impact [8]. Health justice challenges nurses to think beyond the elimination of "health disparities" to a future where resources and power over care technologies like A.I. is more equitably distributed in ways that serve all people, especially those historically and currently excluded from design decision-making.

Consent Most patients and health care workers are familiar with the legal concept of informed consent. The first official use of the term appeared in the 1957 case *Salgo v Leland Stanford Jr. University Board of Trustees*, in which Mr. Salgo sued the university medical center following complications of a contrast agent injection during a cardiovascular assessment which left him partially paralyzed [9]. Mr. Salgo insisted the health system should have disclosed the risk associated with the use of the contrast agent prior to the procedure. At the time of this writing, the USA lacks universal standards for informed consent related to A.I. applications [10]. Ethicists and legal scholars actively debate whether and how patients should be informed about use of A.I. in their care [11]. Traditional clinical consent approaches often include general details about potential benefits and risks of specific medical procedures, but exclude essential details about the role of A.I., related risks, and detailed information on data use and privacy [12]. Debates about procedures for informed consent for A.I. in health care vacillate between clinician-based versus patient-based standards [12]. Clinician-based standards emphasize what a "reasonable" clinician might disclose, while patient-based standards prioritize what patients would most likely want to know. While important, presence of informed consent is a necessary but not sufficient criterion for truly consentful use of A.I [13]. Consent is a dynamic and relational process. The Consentful Tech Project defines "good digital consent" as technology and data systems where permission to apply the technology (or gather, use, archive or share the data it collects) is: Freely-given; Reversible; Informed; Enthusiastic; and Specific [14].

Consent is only possible when refusal is a realistic option. This means patients who decline A.I. use in their care would have other options, including human alternatives. Consentful use of A.I. also implies patients can retract both their consent *and* any data collected by the technology. While policies and practices in most health care settings fall far short of achieving this ideal, nurses have an opportunity to create new systems and technologies that support more consentful use of A.I. in clinical and community care.

Sustainability Nurses have an obligation to engage in sustainable practices that attend to the health of their communities and the planet [15]. Sustainability and planetary health are therefore critical considerations with regard to A.I [16]. While this tech is increasingly applied to a wide array of climate-related challenges, much of the infrastructure that makes A.I. possible generates harmful byproducts while consuming profligate amounts of water, electricity, and other planetary resources [16]. In many areas, A.I. infrastructure such as data centers significantly and negatively impact surrounding communities, driving environmental racism and climate impacts [2]. While more recent technological innovations like chip-level cooling centers may help to mitigate A.I.'s energy footprint, adoption at scale lags behind the accelerating expansion of A.I. data centers and their unprecedented resource demands, placing additional pressures on vital electricity and clean water infrastructure [17]. Large language models (LLMs) that power generative forms of A.I. (like agentic A.I. and ChatGPT) are especially costly with regard to water and electricity consumption, and carbon outputs—though these costs are often deliberately kept secret [2]. At the time of this writing, growing use of generative A.I. represents a severe threat to environmental health and climate futures [16].

A.I. infrastructure's planetary impacts make it difficult, if not impossible, to square further scaling of this tech with nursing's ethics and the pursuit of health justice [18]. When it comes to weighing risks and benefits, nurses face a proximity dilemma. While resource-hungry A.I. may enable better care for individual patients in some circumstances, its accompanying infrastructure is actively harming entire communities and the planet. However, much of the directly observable harm (air pollution, water and electricity consumption, labor exploitation, climate precarity) occurs far from the point of care—while the patient remains directly before them [2, 18]. Nurses practicing in an A.I. era are challenged to engage with these complexities when considering not just how but *whether* use of resource-hungry forms of A.I. are ethical and appropriate.

Invisible Labor Much of the appeal of A.I. in clinical spaces lies in its promise to reduce unnecessary administrative burdens, automate documentation, and assist with other tasks that interfere with nurses' ability to engage directly in patient care [19]. Research to date indicates mixed results with regard to these goals [20]. While A.I. tech may improve efficiency associated with administrative tasks like staff scheduling, documentation or prior authorization, such automation introduces new forms of labor and supervision that may require nurses' time and attention [21]. For example, a recent ethnographic study of an automated sepsis alert system revealed much of the labor nurses engaged in to manage safe use of the A.I., such as assessing and resolving false alarms, was invisible in workflows and undervalued when compared to the A.I. designers' contributions [21]. Meanwhile, some industry actors and health care administrators see A.I. as a path to further reduce staffing shortages and associated costs through the substitution of human health care workers with alternatives such as A.I. agents [22].

If A.I. adoption reduces certain administrative burdens on nurses, but also results in staffing cuts that ultimately reduce the number of human nurses available to care for each patient, do such gains truly serve us? For A.I. to fulfill its promise to improve patient care delivery and outcomes, nurses and health systems will need to attend to both the visible and invisible labor that safe implementation, maintenance, and on-going evaluation of this technology entails [21]. This work will likely require development of new measures of A.I.-related invisible labor, to avoid exacerbating clinician attrition and "burnout" [21]. Nurses must also remain vigilant to impacts of A.I. on their institutions and health care infrastructure, including maintenance of safe and appropriate levels of human staffing, human alternatives to A.I. systems, safety, and care quality [20]. Advocacy for robust contract protections and occupational safety provisions, safe staffing legislation and other state- and federal-level regulations, may help to mitigate impacts of automation on the workforce and patient outcomes.

Generative forms of A.I. (genAI) like OpenAI's ChatGPT and DALL-E often rely on training data collected without the express consent of the persons who originally created it [8]. These training datasets frequently include creative and copyrighted works for which authors might typically expect recognition or financial remuneration. Some forms of genAI train on sensitive data that users might otherwise expect to remain private, such as conversation histories from online therapy platforms. This poses several ethical dilemmas with regard to consent, citation, and privacy. Numerous authors and artists have taken legal action against generative A.I. platforms, alleging theft of their creative works and intellectual property. Some artists have even adopted defensive strategies designed to "poison" A.I. models that make unauthorized use of their work [8]. OpenAI's recent acquisition of the popular learning management system Canvas poses additional ethical questions for nurse educators and learners—as curricular products and homework uploaded to the system is likely to be used to train A.I. models simultaneously being marketed as virtual tutors, care assistants, and educator replacements.

Digital Defense Digital defense represents individual and collective efforts to prevent, protect, and heal from harms associated with technologies that incorporate big data and artificial intelligence [23]. All health technologies (from the scalpel to chemotherapy) are capable of causing harm and *will* cause harm in some contexts, even when applied appropriately [23]. A.I.-related harms range from minor inconveniences (like correcting a typo in the health record made by an auto-scribe) to oppressive and life-threatening consequences (like delivery of an inaccurate assessment from A.I. trained on biased data) [23, 24]. Some of these harms have been well-documented and occur in predictable patterns. Other harms are unpredictable and as yet not fully understood. Often A.I. harms are unevenly distributed, impacting communities already disproportionately impacted by structural oppressions such as racism, poverty, ableism, colonialism, and transphobia [25]. While the existence of harm does not erase possible benefits of some A.I., nurses must be prepared to mitigate (and wherever possible, prevent) harm (see Fig. 6.1).

Imagination for New Futures Although nursing has a long history of health innovation and technological leadership, historical research indicates technologies like A.I. are frequently imposed on nurses and patients, rather than consentfully negotiated [23]. The same can be said for populations whose health and environments are shaped by algorithms and technologies they did not create, nor were ever consulted on—from managed care to credit scores [25]. In order for A.I., or any technology, to help move us closer to health justice, we must first establish the conditions required for consentful use and community control [26]. No one vision of the future is inevitable, nor is the status quo permanent. Creating new and more just futures requires cultivation of a verdant imagination for health care and nursing—understanding not just what is, but what could be. Many A.I. technologies, like large language models (LLMs) and A.I. agents, simply replicate patterns from past data. Some uses of A.I. may help to achieve greater equity and expand access to care. But if we fail to do the creative, relational, human work of imagining and establishing the conditions required for new futures where power over health care and associated technologies is distributed more equitably, widespread A.I. adoption and automation also risks concretizing a fundamentally unjust, chronically understaffed, and segregated health care status quo [23].

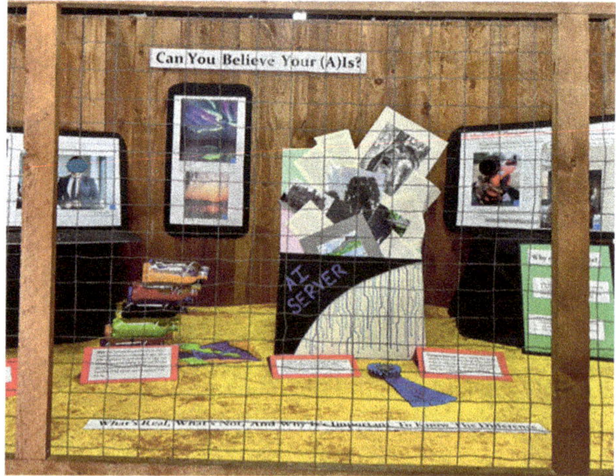

Fig. 6.1 Image credit: "Can you believe your (A) Is?" by Rae Walker

6.3   Impacts of A.I. on Nurses and Nursing Futures

Ensuring patients' safety and well-being is central to nursing's practice so much so, that nurses often neglect their own health and well-being in service of this goal. At the same time, many of the systemic injustices that drive medical errors and health inequities are also rife within the discipline. If we are to create new futures for health justice in an A.I. era, we must first address the injustices that exist within nursing and health care as a whole [26, 27]. Therefore, this chapter's discussion of A.I.'s impacts on clinical care begins with an explanation of how A.I. impacts practicing nurses and nurses' collective well-being.

Nurses do not practice in a vacuum. Figure 6.2 illustrates relationships between A.I. use, nurses, and their environments [23]. We live, work, and play in a socio-technical society where structural and social determinants shape how technologies like A.I. impact care practices and health outcomes. Within this society, governments and state actors apply technologies like A.I. to a myriad of functions in public life—from use of surveillant A.I. like facial recognition cameras to algorithmic systems that manage access to and distribution of social services [29]. Individual institutions, such as hospitals and nursing schools, adopt their own system-wide A.I. These can include technologies like automated worker surveillance and management systems (AWSM), enterprise software that organizes shift schedules, clinical decision support systems (CDSS), resume screeners, or learning management systems. While nurses can make decisions about our personal use of AI tools like ChatGPT, we often have far less control over how and where state- and institutionally-controlled AI applications are applied in our work and daily lives [23].

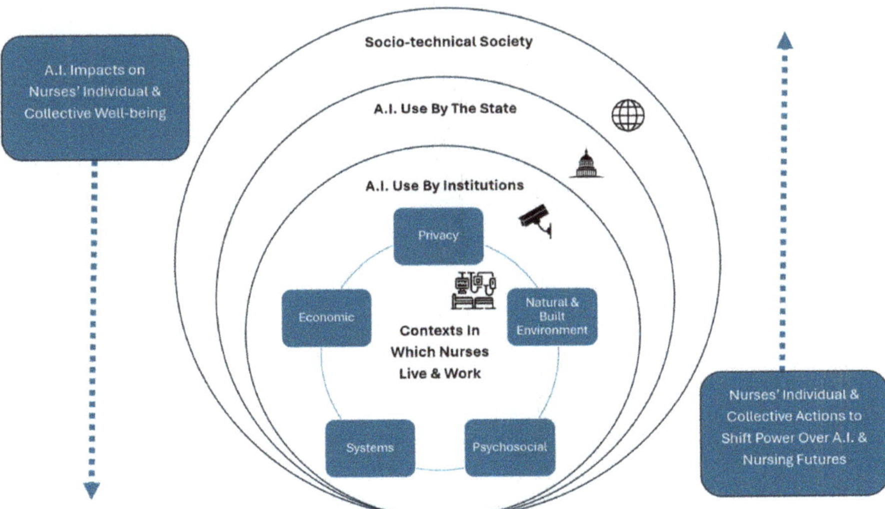

Fig. 6.2 Impacts of Artificial Intelligence on nurses and nursing futures. (Figure adapted with permission by Rae Walker from their framework titled, "A.I. Impacts on Care Workers' Collective Well-being" [23]; originally inspired by the work of Roy and colleagues [28])

Laws, policies, and collective actions like labor strikes shape how and where A.I. use (in society, government, institutions and communities) impact nurses' privacy and the physical, psychosocial, occupational, and economic environments where we live, work, and play. Nurses' social capital (the relational networks built on trust that enable society to function) and collective efficacy (shared beliefs about the ability to achieve desired goals) shape impacts of A.I. on each of these domains. These impacts, filtered through individual nurses' perspectives and actions, affect nurses' collective well-being. This model explains why A.I. can have vastly different impacts on the well-being and care practices of one nurse when compared to another, even as it acts to shape our collective well-being and future.

Collectively, nurses can shape A.I.-related agendas and impacts through development of shared visions for health justice, informed advocacy, and community organizing to support laws and policies that preserve health and human rights [23] (see Fig. 6.3). For example, on March 4, 2025, nurse and Oregon state representative Travis Nelson led successful passage of Oregon's House Bill 2748, which prohibits any "non-human entity" from being called a nurse in that state [30]. The bill was introduced in response to an A.I. company's announcement in spring 2024 that they were poised to introduce a $9/hour "virtual A.I. nurse" [22]. Proponents of the bill were concerned calling the chatbot a "nurse" would result in confusion and loss of

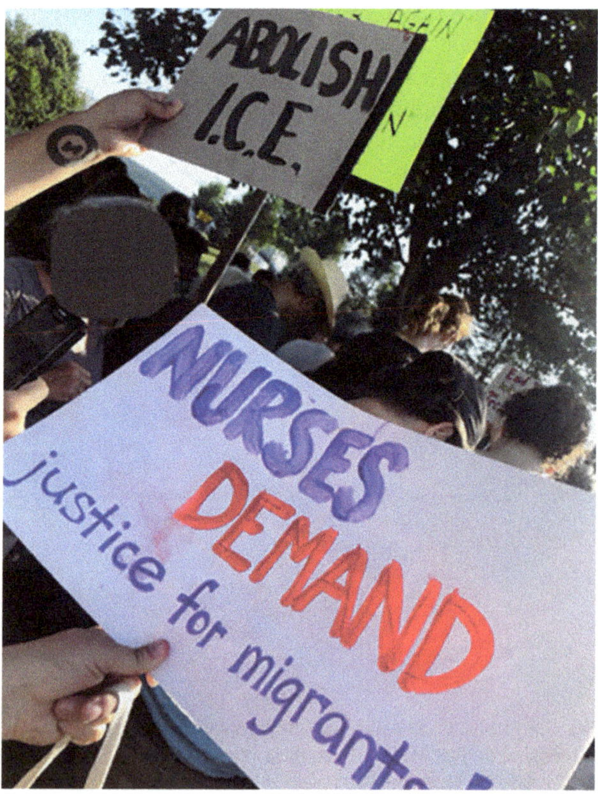

Fig. 6.3 Image credit: "ABOLISH ICE/Nurses demand justice for migrants" by Rae Walker

trust among the public. While the state of Oregon now prohibits the label of "nurse" being applied to non-human entities, most other states lack such legislation.

At the individual level, nurses make choices about our own behaviors and care practices. These can include choices like assisting in the design of new algorithmic systems, conducting research on A.I. and its impacts, advocating for institutional and governmental policies that support more consentful use of A.I. technologies, and refusing technologies and data regimes that cause harm. Consent cannot exist unless the possibility of refusal, without coercion or retaliation, is a real option. Refusal is a type of digital defense that may take the form of:

- Abstaining from use of a certain technology in favor of a human alternative (for example, a nurse who refuses to use genAI in their writing process).
- Selecting a *different* technology that is more ethically sound, sustainable, safer or efficacious (such as using a secure web browser that does not include web trackers that can siphon off sensitive information).
- Calls to action (such as leading a public health advocacy campaign to resist unregulated expansion of power-hungry data centers).
- Whistleblowing to report and prevent further harm.

Nurse Advocacy for Consentful Data Practices

Policy advocacy is an important form of nursing practice that in turn shapes clinical care. In the spring of 2024, I was asked to provide expert testimony about A.I. for health care to a federal committee focused on creating a strategic plan for the future of health information technology in the United States. My testimony as a Registered Nurse led to an invitation to join a federal rules advisory task force organized by a group known as the Health Information Technology Advisory Committee (HITAC).

When Congress passes legislation, it must designate groups of people to design the rules that will determine exactly how that legislation will be enacted. When the twenty-first Century Cures Act was enacted in 2016, the legislation demanded creation of a national health records database. Health systems that receive federal funds (including from Medicare and Medicaid) are now required to share de-identified data from their EHRs with the U.S. government. This is a significant shift in how health data are handled. The law has many implications for public health and privacy.

As a nurse inventor and researcher who studies data and power, I know this national EHR database could help promote health equity (for example, by enabling faster detection of trends that might benefit from policy and public health interventions). However, the database could also expose the health histories of entire communities—introducing new potentials for data abuse, privacy violations, and bias. In a world where datasets are increasingly combined, no dataset is ever truly 'de-identified'. Since these data will likely be used to train new forms of A.I., they could have a significant influence well into the future.

(continued)

In our current political climate, some forms of health care are increasingly criminalized at the state and federal levels. This means mandated data-sharing with the federal government could have unintended and negative consequences which are likely to impact groups already adversely affected by power inequities. However, according to the legislation, EHR data pertaining to patients' reproductive health care are protected from having to be automatically shared. And the rules determining what 'counted' as protected reproductive health data. So I used my nursing knowledge to advocate for the rule to include the broadest possible interpretation of what constitutes reproductive health data. I did this so individual clinics and communities could exercise greater autonomy when making decisions about how and whether to share data that could potentially be weaponized against both patients and care workers.

Many of our efforts to protect data-related civil rights and patient privacy at the federal level were overturned when a new presidential administration transitioned into power in 2025. I continue to apply my nursing knowledge to advocate for privacy and more consentful tech, including at city council meetings within my community. Relationship-building and nursing practice at the local level is just as (if not even more!) necessary as efforts to shift federal and state policy.—RW.

6.4 A.I. in Clinical Care

Many of the technologies that currently fall under the "A.I." umbrella have long been an established part of the clinical environment. This is especially true in relation to analytical approaches like machine learning, and tools like wearable sensors used in continuous patient monitoring, transcription software, and certain automated features in the electronic health record. Adoption of new forms of A.I. into clinical care continues to accelerate, with many products now called A.I. whether or not they meet traditional definitions of the term [8]. Research indicates tech start-ups whose products include the label "A.I." receive 15–50% more money from investors [31]. This phenomenon of labeling non-A.I. products A.I. to enhance their marketability is known as "A.I.-washing."

Researchers have created consensus-based guidelines and tools like the "REFORMS" checklist to aid clinicians and consumers in discerning which technologies are actually A.I. and judging the quality of evidence to support their use [3]. Model cards are another recent innovation designed to improve A.I. transparency, explainability, and safety. First proposed by A.I. ethics researcher Margaret Mitchell, and fashioned after analog technologies like nutrition labels, model cards provide clinicians and patients with information about the intended function of an A.I. model, how it was designed and by whom, metrics of accuracy and uncertainty, and performance across representative and intersectional populations [32]. The Coalition for Health A.I. (www.chai.org) developed a template for A.I. model cards in health care. A version of this template was released under a Creative Commons license (CC BY-NC-ND 4.0) for public comment in November 2024, and is currently under on-going evaluation. The template is organized according to CHAI's Five Principles of Responsible A.I.: Transparency, Safety, Security & Privacy, Fairness & Bias, and Usefulness. More information including detailed instructions for use and completed examples can be accessed at: https://www.chai.org/workgroup/applied-model

Nurses should be ready to encounter a wide variety of A.I. applications whose presence and function may not always be transparent, even with a model card. These include applications to continuous patient monitoring and predictive analytics, nursing assessment and diagnostics, clinical decision support, documentation, interprofessional collaboration, care delivery, patient education, workflow management, and worker surveillance. Though the A.I. landscape continues to change rapidly, familiarizing yourself with common forms of clinical A.I. and how they function will help prepare you to critically assess and communicate potential benefits and risks to patients, communities, and the planet. Table 6.1 provides an overview and examples of A.I. applications across the continuum of care.

Table 6.1 A.I. Across the continuum of care

Stage of care continuum	Care category	Description	Example
Prevention and wellness	Preventive care	Numerous A.I. technologies are in development to assist with screening for conditions such as breast cancer and cognitive syndromes. Some of these approaches involve chatbots, while others integrate LLMs or computer vision to analyze results. Increasingly, companies are using A.I.-enabled tools to identify and target consumers who might be likely to use their commercially-available screening products. As more and more care interactions are digitally recorded and archived, patients will need to develop greater awareness of when and how their data may be used and shared. For example, a patient who is an immigrant and seeks counseling from a chatbot may be exposed to risk of legal consequences if that company shares their data with agencies like Immigration and Customs Enforcement (ICE), as recently happened with some immigrants' Medicaid data. A patient who resides in a state where abortion care access has been criminalized may be harmed if sensitive data from their period tracker is shared with state authorities. Nurses must also attend to their own A.I.-enabled documentation practices, to ensure data are recorded accurately and consentfully. New forms of A.I.-enabled screening raise new questions about data use, consent, and patient privacy [33]. One such example is "voice biomarkers" that screen patient voice recordings for signs of illness or cognitive decline. While intended to help, such tools—when applied non-consensually—have significant potential for weaponization and abuse.	DermaSensor recently became the first A.I.-powered tool to be approved by the FDA for diagnosis of skin cancer, including melanoma, basal cell carcinoma, and squamous cell carcinoma. The tool is designed to be used non-invasively at the point of care by primary care providers who may not have the same level of dermatological expertise as a specialist. Its approval follows an observational study involving >1000 patients at the Mayo Clinic. The sample included patients with a diverse range of skin conditions and pigmentation levels [34].
	Wellness	A.I. has a growing role in the wellness industry. Wearable devices like smart watches and ambient intelligence like smart speakers can provide instant access to a wide variety of programs offering virtual services like exercise classes, dietary and cooking advice, health coaching, guided meditation, counseling, and self-improvement. Data collected by these devices is not necessarily protected by privacy laws like HIPAA [3]. Data collected by many of these devices may be shared or sold to other companies, impacting user privacy. Companies also use consumers' data (including datasets purchased from data brokers) to target and persuade individuals to purchase their products via personalized advertisements.	Consumer-grade augmented reality (AR) and virtual reality (VR) gaming systems provide an engaging and immersive environment on-demand. One study of the use of Oculus VR System among persons managing Parkinson's indicated the platform provided a safe means to boost patients' working memory and mood in the home setting [35].

| Access to care | Access to care | Telehealth services and private health technology start-ups have expanded health care access in some health care "deserts." Tech such as genAI chatbots and A.I. agents promise to further expand care to individuals who are unable to access in-person health care services and those who find such services do not meet their health needs. However, such tools have significant limitations. They cannot replace human relationships or the full scope of human health care workers' capability. For example, A.I. agents cannot provide hands-on care. App-ified health services offered by private vendors may not necessarily take insurance, and data shared via these platforms may not be subject to the same privacy protections required by HIPAA. Some communities impacted by the "digital divide" may experience less access to health care as the current human health care infrastructure is replaced with virtual alternatives. Others may worry about possible legal and privacy consequences of sharing their information via digital platforms [3]. | Crisis text line is a well-established non-profit that manages a mental health support line. The non-profit caused controversy when it was revealed that it shared data from patient encounters with a private A.I. start-up, raising questions about privacy and safety [36]. A study of human crisis hotline workers' perspectives on A.I. integration revealed that while some were hopeful A.I. technology could be helpful, they also expressed concerns about A.I. inflexibility, emotional safety, and potentials for dehumanization of callers in distress [37]. |
| | Prior authorizations | Insurance companies increasingly rely on A.I. automation to review and process claims and requests for prior authorization (PA). A 2024 survey conducted by the American Medical Association indicated 61% of physicians fear payers' use of unregulated AI is increasing PA denials [38]. Investigative journalists have revealed these fears are likely founded, as payers use algorithms to enable mass denial of PA requests in order to boost profits [29]. While insurance providers are required to keep human providers in the loop, many have found work arounds [3]. At the same time, some clinical centers have begun relying on A.I.-enabled services to expedite and improve success rates obtaining PAs for their patients. | At a large academic medical center in the Boston region, nurses have enlisted the services of an A.I.-enabled private agency to off-load administrative burdens associated with obtaining prior authorizations from insurance companies. Nurses report anecdotal evidence that patients receive more timely approvals, while nurses have more time to spend on other aspects of patient care. |

(continued)

Table 6.1 (continued)

Stage of care continuum	Care category	Description	Example
Support for clinical decision-making and care transitions	Diagnostics	Most of the currently approved diagnostic forms of clinical A.I. are designed for use by providers with prescribing privileges [39]. Some of these tools have already impacted care for high stakes medical scenarios such as stroke. In some cases, introduction of diagnostic A.I. has changed clinical workflows. As of this writing, A.I. technology is not allowed to *independently* diagnose or prescribe in the USA. In 2025, U.S. Representative Schweikert introduced a bill that would allow the FDA to redefine "prescriber" to include A.I. Should such legislation be adopted, we will likely see expansion of diagnostic applications marketed directly to consumers via commercial platforms like social media. Research on clinician use of some forms of A.I. support in clinical assessment suggests high levels of use may be associated with reductions in clinicians' capacity for critical reasoning [40]. These findings and other recent events, such as the widespread "Crowdstrike" outage that disabled many health systems' computers in July 2024, point to the importance of nurses maintaining clinical knowledge and analog skills in addition to developing technological competency.	Both patients and clinicians are increasingly turning to resources like LLMs to provide diagnostic guidance. However, LLMs rely heavily on whatever training data they are exposed to, which can contain inaccuracies and bias [29]. A recent single-blind randomized controlled trial of LLM (ChatGPT 4.0) use among 50 physicians found its use did not improve clinicians' diagnostic accuracy [41]. Health systems should also consider planetary costs and exercise tremendous caution when incorporating A.I. automation for diagnostic guidance.
	Predictive analytics	A.I. applications for predictive analytics typically analyze information in the electronic health record to provide early warnings about patient risk or deterioriation, or to forecast resource demands and coordinate systems-level response [19]. Some of the applications are well-established, but most remain under development. Systems to predict risk of sepsis and falls are some of the most common applications, and widely integrated across many EHRs and clinical settings [21]. Nursing care associated with these systems includes responding to alerts, conducting further patient assessment and coordinating interventions, when appropriate [42]. We do not yet have enough research to state whether predictive analytics reduce or exacerbate burden and alarm fatigue, though some ethnographic research suggests these systems can entail considerable invisible labor by nurses [20, 21].	The Communicating Narrative Concerns Entered by RNs (CONCERN) study is a recent multi-site trial that tested predictive monitoring technology designed to provide hospital staff with early warnings of patient deterioration. Over 60,000 hospital encounters, risk of instantaneous death was reduced by 35.6% among patients in the intervention group. Use of the machine learning application was also associated with decreased length of stay, decreased risk of sepsis, and increased risk of instantaneous transfer to the ICU [43].
	Assessing patient acuity	Automated patient acuity scoring draws on information in electronic health records (EHR) systems to determine how much care a patient may require. These calculations impact patient triage, nurse staffing levels and patient assignments. Nursing unions like National Nurses United have gone on strike to protest loss of nursing autonomy with regard to their ability to exercise clinical judgment. In a recent survey of more than 2000 California nurses, many reported differences between their own assessments and automated acuity scores that could not be changed in the EHR [44].	The Cleveland Clinic command center analyzes automated acuity scores and other data from across their health system to coordinate dynamic staff scheduling in response to predicted shifts in demand. The Cleveland Clinic command center analyzes automated acuity scores and other data from across their health system to coordinate dynamic staff scheduling in response to predicted shifts in demand [45].
	Symptom management	AI approaches such as machine learning (ML) and natural language processing (NLP) have already been applied to the nursing management of a wide range of symptoms such as pain, psychological distress, nausea, vomiting, and fatigue. For some patients and caregivers, A.I.-powered chatbots are a convenient, on-demand addition to their supportive care team. This aligns with prior research indicating some patients prefer to interact with non-human platforms when seeking information and support, while others continue to prefer human-delivered A.I. alternatives. When it comes to symptom management, there is no such thing as a "one-size-fits-all" solution.	ChemoFreeBot is a chatbot designed to converse with patients receiving chemotherapy, offering personalized symptom support and education. In one study, participants who interacted with ChemoFreeBot reported significantly lower frequencies and severity of physical and psychological symptoms compared with those in a nurse-led education group or routine care [46].
	Care planning and discharge	A.I. tools like predictive analytics are being used to help determine when it's safe for a patient to undergo a care transition such as discharge from the hospital. By analyzing information from the EHR using approaches like neural networks, these AI models are designed to help identify who is ready for discharge and who might need to stay longer for extra care. Such technology may help reduce risk by avoiding sending patients home too early, while reducing length of stay when appropriate [47]. At the same time, some algorithms applied to hospital discharge planning have been shown to amplify dangerous biases as a result of historical patterns in their training data, such as medical racism [24]. Resource-hungry genAI tools like ChatGPT are also being explored for generating nursing care plans and discharge summaries. While these tools may help reduce nurses' administrative burden, thorough human oversight is always necessary to ensure care plans are safe, individualized, and clinically appropriate.	In one external validation study conducted in the Netherlands, the DESIRE A.I. tool was retrospectively analyzed using post-surgical patient data from hundreds of patient encounters. The best-performing version of the model had a negative predictive value (NPV) of 89.3%. Researchers hypothesize application of the model might help to conserve hospital resources and reduce risks of post-operative complications, though further testing is needed to establish its efficacy in other environments [47].

Evaluation of care outcomes	Continuous and remote patient monitoring	A.I.-integrated remote patient monitoring collects and analyzes real-time data from wearables (like smart watches, rings and skin patches) and environmental sensors (like smart speakers, video cameras, and wall-mounted radar), implantable medical devices, and patient-reported outcomes. Some of these sensors send data one-way, directly to the clinician or EHR. Some are designed to provide data displays and alerts directly to patients and informal or remote caregivers. Many of these devices require use of proprietary software and hardware, requiring patients to agree to terms of service that include sharing sensitive data such as their health information, location, or video and audio recordings with private companies in ways that fall outside of the typical privacy protections of HIPAA.	For patients using neuromodulation therapies, such as spinal cord stimulation, A.I.-integrated remote patient monitoring (RPM) enables clinicians to receive continuous or on-demand feedback on therapy usage, device performance, and patient-reported pain outcomes. Such information may help to support proactive clinical decisions and improve patient safety [48].
	Detecting racism and bias in care	Nurse researchers have begun developing tools to detect and address racism and other forms of bias in nursing care. Some of these tools rely on natural language processing applications embedded in EHR systems to analyze nursing notes for biased and stigmatizing language. Nurse researchers have also developed interventions that use VR to promote development of interracial empathy and reduce bias through immersive learning experiences involving avatars [49].	The NIH-funded ENGAGE study led by principal investigator Maxim Topaz of Columbia University alongside co-PIs Scott M. Sittig and Jacquelyn Y. Taylor aims to develop an NLP-driven system to rEduce stigmatiziNG languAGE (ENGAGE) used in home health care clinical notes.
Care for populations and the planet	Addressing social and structural determinants of health (SDOH)	Some A.I. applications address SDOH such as housing insecurity and homelessness, neighborhood and built environment, income and socioeconomic status, employment, family and social support, food insecurity, insurance status and stability, and history of incarceration. A common example is health information exchanges (HIE) that promote the simultaneous sharing and tracking of patient data and trends across multiple organizations and disparate datasets. State and local agencies also rely on A.I. automation to administer many social services programs, sometimes with biased results [29]. The gravity project is a nurse-engaged public collaboration that develops consensus-based data standards, such as ICD-10 codes, to improve incorporation of data on social need and social determinants of health into systems that provide clinical and community-based care. While these data standards may provide important benefits, widespread collection of such data introduces new surveillance and data privacy concerns, especially when data are shared with state actors and across multiple platforms.	ThriveLink is an ANA innovation award-winning A.I.-powered platform that provides telephonic support for enrollment in social services and programs like WIC, SNAP, and Medicaid. It was created by a nurse manager named Kwamane Liddell, to help prevent patients from being kicked off Medicaid. The company claims use of the platform reduces staff workloads associated with paper forms. Bilingual (Spanish/English) community health workers remain in the loop to assist when needed.
	Disaster and climate crisis preparation and response	A.I. designed to predict trends (in weather, infectious disease, mortality and other phenomena) related to a changing climate, or to aid in preparation for and response to associated disasters such as disease outbreaks, wildfires, flash floods, and heat waves. While some A.I. may aid in climate resilience, many A.I. applications simultaneously consume considerable electricity, water, and other non-renewable resources, thus increasing climate volatility [16].	A.I.-enabled wildfire modelling has been deployed during recent large wildfires, such as those which occurred in Los Angeles in 2025, to help determine fire spread and severity, so warnings could be sent and resources could be triaged appropriately.
	Public health surveillance	Some A.I. applications scan patterns across the internet (ex. social media, government agencies, news, local observers) to detect outbreaks and other shifts in population health, predict trends, continuously monitor and assess outcomes.	SENTINEL is software that uses deep neural networks to scan social media, news, and clinical sources to provide health officials with early warnings, situational awareness and "now-casting" (disease prediction) [50].

6.5   Clinical Decision-Making Support (CDSS)

A.I. technologies are increasingly embedded into clinical decision-making support for health care staff and the patients they accompany in care. A.I. use in CDSS has grown exponentially in recent years and is expected to continue to expand in areas such as patient monitoring and predictive analytics, diagnostics, care-planning, and symptom management. By the time this text is printed just a few months from now, even more applications will have likely been introduced. Some CDSS systems have been extensively researched, while others are just emerging [39]. Laws and institutional policies that regulate uses of A.I. shape what uses are approved for use in formal health care settings. While several systems are already widely integrated, many more are currently being researched but not yet approved for wider use in patient care. Far fewer have been externally validated across diverse settings and datasets, limiting how much we can conclude about their safety, efficacy, and acceptability across diverse clinical contexts and patient populations [51].

Some CDSS show great promise to improve health outcomes and health equity, including for patient populations commonly excluded from clinical research—like neonates, pregnant persons, and children [42]. However in many cases, CDSS have yet to fully live up to developers' claims—a phenomenon known as "A.I. hype" [8]. In order to provide patients with clear and accurate information about the risks and benefits of CDSS, nurses must separate A.I. hype from reality [8]. Nurse informaticists can assist this process by auditing clinical algorithms to assess their performance and bias. AI model cards and publicly available guidelines (like those from the Coalition for Health A.I. or Obermeyer and colleagues' Algorithmic Bias Playbook) can assist in the generation of robust and comparable data about the clinical performance of A.I. systems. Nurses at the bedside must take care to critically consider CDSS products. While such tools may help reduce some of the cognitive load on the nurse, nurses must continue to use their expert clinical judgment to maintain oversight and better ensure safe application of CDSS outputs.

6.6   Patient Monitoring and Predictive Analytics

A.I.-enabled patient monitoring and predictive analytics leverage vast amounts of patient data to forecast future health events, trends, and resource needs (see Table 6.2). Some of these tools have potential to provide critical insights that may enhance clinical decision-making, allowing nurses to proactively intervene and implement timely and targeted interventions [42]. Predictive analytics support patient-centered care by enabling development of individualized care plans based on analyses of data about patients' current therapies and health history, social needs, lifestyle, genomics, and environment. Some research has demonstrated integration of predictive models into clinical workflows can reduce the prevalence of hospital-acquired pressure injuries and improve fall prevention [39]. However, fewer than 4% of studies of clinical A.I. published in high-impact health informatics journals in the last 13 years have validated their models using datasets other than the original

Table 6.2 A.I.-enabled predictive analytics examples with nursing considerations

Nursing care focus: prevention of pressure injuries in critical care

Example of an A.I. Application
Bayesian network is an A.I. system developed using EHR data from patients on the intensive care unit. The model incorporates information such as patients' medication use, diagnoses, and Braden scale scores to predict the risk of developing pressure ulcers. The model constructs a visual representation of risks that allows clinicians to work proactively to prevent pressure ulcers by identifying persons at higher risk early before a problem develops [53].

Evidence of impact
Much of the published research on pressure injury prediction in ICU consists of modeling studies that demonstrate high predictive accuracy but do not report intervention outcomes. However, a pre-post experimental study showed use of the Bayesian network model was associated with a clinically significant reduction in hospital-acquired pressure injuries, with prevalence dropping from 21% at baseline to 4% post-intervention [53]. The average ICU length of stay decreased from 7.6 to 5.2 days.

Key nursing considerations

Consent	Health justice	Sustainability	Invisible labor	Digital defense
A.I. systems for pressure injury prevention often function in the background, analyzing data without direct patient interaction. This raises concerns about *informed consent and transparency. For example:* If an AI model flags a patient as high risk for pressure injuries, leading to more frequent repositioning or special mattress use, the patient should be informed that this care is guided in part by predictive algorithms.	A.I. models may *perpetuate or even exacerbate health inequities* if they are trained on biased or incomplete data. *For example:* An AI model trained primarily on data from individuals with lighter skin tones might fail to identify pressure injury risks in patients with darker skin tones, placing them at greater risk for harm.	A.I. models must be *continuously updated, validated, and monitored* to ensure they remain clinically relevant and accurate over time. Changes in clinical practice, patient populations, or documentation standards can all affect A.I. performance. *For example:* A model developed pre-pandemic may not account for new patient care patterns seen in COVID-era ICU settings, requiring revalidation.	While A.I. systems aim to assist clinicians, they can unintentionally add to *nurses' workload* through increased documentation demands, frequent alerts, or the need to verify AI-generated recommendations. *For example:* An algorithm that continually sends up alerts for pressure injury may require a nurse to step away from other duties to perform a focused assessment, whether or not the alert is accurate or appropriate. When not appropriately accounted for in nursing's workflows, such alerts can contribute to alarm fatigue and burnout.	A.I. systems handle sensitive health information, making *data privacy and cybersecurity* essential. In order to fully communicate the safety and risks of A.I. systems to patients, nurses must understand how patient data is stored, shared, and used by AI tools. While technological surveillance is common in many acute care settings, the scope and capability of these tools is rapidly expanding. *For example:* Facial recognition software, in particular, poses specific risks not only to patients but also visitors and anyone whose presence may be tracked and shared without their express knowledge and consent.

(continued)

Table 6.2 (continued)

Nursing care focus: Falls prevention

Example of an A.I. Application

Machine learning algorithms and deep learning approaches—such as gradient boosting machines and extreme gradient boosting (XGBoost)—are frequently used to develop predictive models for patient fall risk based on clinical data. These models are currently used across multiple settings including in the home, community, and hospitals. One example is an XGBoost model that was developed using patients' gait features to predict their fall risk. In this study, fall risk was categorized into high- and low-risk groups. Across all walking speeds, the model identified three gait features—Stride length, walking speed, and stance phase—as key predictors of fall risk [54].

Evidence of impact

Current research provides promising evidence that A.I. models can accurately predict fall risk in some settings and patient populations, especially for older adults. In one recent systematic review, all fall prediction models demonstrated accuracy levels of over 70% [39]. The XGBoost model was more sensitive than the Morse fall scale, and a comparative study showed that the A.I. prediction model was comparable to traditional models for assessing fall risk. However, nurses reviewing research on A.I. model performance should keep in mind that such research is rarely externally validated [52]. This means while the research may report high levels of model accuracy, A.I. Models may perform far less well or predictably when applied in a new setting, with new patients, or over time.

Key nursing considerations

Consent	Health justice	Sustainability	Invisible labor	Digital defense
AI-powered fall prediction models often use patient data from EHRs, sensors, or wearable devices to assess risk—frequently without *explicit patient consent* for each use. *For example:* Patients should be informed if fall risk scores are generated from wearable gait sensors, bed alarms, or other surveillant technologies that use AI to classify risk level.	All A.I. models contain potential for *algorithmic bias* (systematic errors that create inequitable, unfair, and/or harmful outcomes associated with human biases present in the training data, design or use of the model). *For example:* Adults who use assistive devices (e.g., walkers) or who have non-standard gait patterns due to injuries, differences in body morphology, or neurological conditions, may be misclassified by a model whose training data did not include such forms of diversity.	A.I. fall prevention systems require *external validation, ongoing evaluation and recalibration* to remain effective across different care settings and patient populations. *For example:* A predictive model developed in a hospital setting may not function well for community-dwelling older adults unless it is retrained using representative and intersectional community-based data.	A.I.-generated fall risk scores or alerts can create additional responsibilities for nurses, including *reviewing alerts, reassessing patients, or implementing added precautions*. This labor must be accounted for in clinical workflows, patient assignments, and nurse staffing levels. *For example:* Automated alert systems may generate false alarms, disrupting nurses' workflow and taking them away from other patient care responsibilities.	Fall prediction tools must be *secure, auditable, and explainable,* especially when linked to sensitive data or surveillance like sensor-based movement tracking or video monitoring. *For example:* If the A.I. relies on commercially available technologies like smart watches or in-home cameras, patients may need to review their privacy and security settings to better protect their data from unintended or criminal use.

training data [52]. Many developers rely on the same open source EHR datasets (like MIMIC and eICU) to build their A.I. models. This creates the possibility of "over-fitting"—creating models that work well with their original training data (which they were built on), but poorly or unpredictably when applied to other settings where the data are not such a close match. A recent critical review of predictive A.I. in critical care concluded widespread failure of peer-reviewed journals to require external validation of A.I. models is a threat to responsible research and the generalizability of research findings [52]. Use of "black box" algorithms and lack of universal A.I. labeling standards and associated transparency about model functioning present barriers to safe and consentful application of these technologies [14]. Nurses should continue to use their clinical judgment to continually assess patients' goals, needs, and condition, remaining vigilant for changes.

6.7   Diagnostics

A.I.-enabled technologies are becoming an increasingly common addition to clinicians' diagnostic toolkits [39] (see Table 6.3). Some health systems already incorporate A.I. to identify patients who might develop serious complications, so care teams can better anticipate and prevent such outcomes and unnecessary readmissions. A.I. may also help by warning about medication risks, taking into account an individual's care regimen, health history, lifestyle, social needs, and omic profile, so they can make more informed decisions about their care [39]. User-friendly A.I. programs with intuitive interfaces may help support nurses' use of their expert clinical judgment to assess patient needs, identify underlying problems, recommend therapeutic approaches, and engage in delivery of patient education and clinical care. Increasingly available agentic A.I. systems are designed to support telehealth delivery and real-time, data-informed decision-making. Appropriate and consentful integration of such A.I. tools could help to reduce certain health inequities [19]. As telehealth delivery continues to evolve alongside A.I., it has the potential to make diagnostic support and timely health care more widely available. However, this potential will only be realized if the social, political, and environmental conditions required for equitable, safe, and consentful application of these technologies are established and maintained [14].

Coded biases in algorithm design and training data mean A.I. diagnostic tools do not serve everyone equitably. Generative A.I. diagnostics often rely on LLMs that reinforce existing biases and misconceptions, like incorrect and racist assumptions about race-based biological differences. Groups more likely to be harmed by algorithmic biases include anyone currently and historically excluded from training datasets and A.I. design decision-making [25]. Nurses need to be aware of these limitations, which should inform their care, communication with patients, and consent practices. Wherever possible, nurses should advocate for diverse, representative and intersectional design teams and training datasets, reparative practices to address structural biases, and clear and transparent labeling and oversight of A.I. tools' design and functioning.

Table 6.3 A.I. in diagnostics examples with nursing considerations

Nursing care focus: patient assessment via telehealth

Examples of A.I. Applications

An A.I. agent is a system or program that is capable of autonomously performing tasks on behalf of a user or another system by designing its workflow and utilizing available tools. Unlike genAI like ChatGPT, agentic A.I. does not require specific prompts from the user to take action. A.I. agents are currently being developed to engage in clinical assessment and decision making, patient education, and delivery of dialogue-based therapeutic interventions like motivational interviewing. When necessary, some A.I. agents can interact with external systems to communicate information or initiate referrals. Nurses may encounter A.I. agent used by their health systems—to assist with tasks such as managing queries in the patient portal, patient education, and some forms of standardized screening and assessment. Nurses may also be tasked with monitoring these interactions or caring for patients referred by the A.I. agent.

AMIE (articulate medical intelligence expert) is a conversational diagnostic A.I. system designed to simulate the clinical reasoning and dialogue of a human clinician. AMIE's model is refined through supervised learning, self-play, and expert feedback. The model gathers relevant clinical information through text-based patient exchanges, formulates differential diagnoses (DDx), and suggests possible care approaches.

Evidence of impacts

The AMIE chatbot imitates a human clinician during patient interviews conducted via telehealth. The A.I. agent engages patients in multi-turn conversations. In experiments involving simulated patients, AMIE's performance was rated higher than some human primary care providers on certain measures of diagnostic accuracy and empathy. This system was recently evaluated in a multi-site randomized cross-over trial conducted in Canada, the U.K. and India.

AMIE is similar to other agentic A.I. tools already available on the market, such as Hippocratic A.I.'s "A.I. virtual nurse" [37]. Hippocratic A.I.'s technology also relies on a cluster of LLMs, each of which are trained to perform different tasks (such as imitating empathic bedside manner, analyzing patient lab values, administering routine screening tools, or providing motivational interviewing for lifestyle adaptation). The Hippocratic A.I. agent webstore went live in spring 2025 and currently features hundreds of A.I. agents. At the time of this writing, however, results of experiments involving Hippocratic A.I.'s virtual care assistants have been reported primarily by the company, rather than independently verified through peer-reviewed research. While numerous nurses have been involved in the development and evaluation of the technology, lack of independent external review severely limits how much we can conclude about its safety, efficacy, and acceptability.

(continued)

Table 6.3 (continued)

Key nursing considerations				
Consent	**Health justice**	**Sustainability**	**Invisible labor**	**Digital defense**
Some A.I. agents are available in multiple languages, potentially improving delivery of consentful care. However, integration of AI into clinical diagnosis also poses risks, such as the possibility of algorithmic bias that leads to errors. The "*black box*" nature of many systems undermines transparency and patient trust.	Due to *structural oppressions* like racism that impact both training datasets and who gets to design and control A.I., models may be more likely to underdiagnose or misdiagnose conditions among persons excluded from or under-represented in the training data, and among persons historically subjected to diagnostic biases.	Using agentic A.I. for assessment and diagnosis requires large amounts of *electricity and water, increased carbon emissions*, and possible generation of *harmful byproducts* that have poisoned some communities. These changes may also contribute to public health problems through added *pollution, climate impacts, and environmental racism*. Although such impacts are often deliberately kept secret, nurses should keep such costs in mind when evaluating the ethics of A.I. use.	When A.I. is applied to assessment and diagnosis, nurses continue to do a lot of important work behind the scenes (known as *invisible labor*). They help prepare and check the accuracy of data used by the system, find and address mistakes, and translate A.I.-generated outputs into actual patient care. They also help their teams learn to use these new tools and supervise their use. Even though this work is vitally important, it is not always valued or accounted for in clinical workflows, promotion structures, or paychecks.	Integration of A.I. into healthcare diagnostics has improved the speed and accuracy of diagnoses for some patients. However, these results are not universal. A.I. systems require access to large amounts of sensitive health data, leading to increased *cybersecurity risks like data breaches and cyberattacks*. These risks threaten patient privacy and can disrupt healthcare services, as seen in major incidents like the 2024 change healthcare cyberattack. It's important to balance the potential benefits of A.I. with strong cybersecurity measures to protect both patients and healthcare providers from harm and to maintain trust in digital healthcare systems.

6.8   Collaboration and Team-Based Care

A.I. has become a common feature of clinical communication platforms like EHRs, clinic scheduling platforms, and automated worker surveillance and management systems (AWSM). Many email and messaging platforms now integrate A.I. tools to summarize and prioritize messages. Much nurse-patient communication has now moved online via telehealth and electronic patient portals. NLP and LLMs have been applied to help streamline and triage growing numbers of patient messages and queries. Researchers are now testing A.I. models designed to detect and act on patient messages that contain information that indicates possible need for an urgent response [55]. Some health systems are also piloting new strategies like telemedicine-enhanced team-based care models that use A.I. to help to anticipate specific patient needs and tailor individualized care plans that draw on multidisciplinary expertise.

6.9   Workflow Optimization and Digital Worker Surveillance

A.I.-enabled continuous monitoring applies not only to patients, but increasingly, to health care workers themselves via AWSM systems. For example, calendar applications like Nurse Grid allow nurses and nurse managers to see everyone else who is assigned to work their shifts, communicate scheduling preferences, and organize shift swaps and vacation days. While some of these systems have been designed with the purpose of optimizing clinical workflows and reducing clinician "burn-out," nursing unions like National Nurses United have expressed concern about potential impacts of automated digital surveillance on nurses' privacy, autonomy, and ability to organize [44]. Nursing scholars like Jess Dillard-Wright have noted how even EHRs serve as a sort of digital panopticon, structuring delivery of nursing care through rigid lists of tasks and disciplining nurses whose documentation fails to conform or check every box within the allotted window [56]. In 2023, the White House Office of Science and Technology Policy requested public comment on impacts of AWSM in the workplace. The Government Accountability Office reviewed public comments submitted by workers, researchers, labor representatives, trade associations, and advocacy organizations. Respondents noted employers used a variety of digital surveillance tools to track workers' location and productivity, including cameras and microphones, geolocation and tracking applications, and devices worn by workers (such as RFID tags). Many respondents expressed concern over privacy and lack of transparency with regard to how worker data was used and shared. Some respondents suggested ubiquitous monitoring negatively impacted worker morale by decreasing trust and possibly discouraging union organizing.

6.10   A.I. and Gig Nursing

A.I. is foundational to many aspects of the so-called gig economy, and nursing is no exception. Some tech start-ups have capitalized on COVID-era clinical workforce shortages and the rise of travel nursing by offering apps that allow nurses to bid for and schedule individual shifts at different clinical sites. These tools allow health care centers to advertise shift vacancies, along with information such as required skills and certifications. Apps like Gale and ShiftMed allow nurses to view available shifts in their area and indicate which ones they are interested in. Sometimes nurses must bid on shifts by indicating their desired rate of pay. Not unlike online shopping platforms like eBay, unit managers can then view all the bids and select the nurse they wish to cover the shift. While this may provide a more flexible scheduling option for some nurses, the "gig-ification" of nursing has implications for patient and nurse safety, unit morale and team-based care. A recent tech policy brief on this rising phenomenon, dubbed "Uber for nursing," highlighted serious concerns including that such apps encourage nurses to work for less pay, do not provide certainty with regard to the amount of work or timing, have little accountability for users' well-being, and may threaten patient safety by placing nurses in unfamiliar clinical environments without any on-boarding, clinical supervision, or facility-specific training [57].

6.11   Conclusions and Future Directions

Creating new futures for nursing in an A.I. era, while staying true to nursing's ethics and social contract, will require continuously analyzing and recommitting to each other, our communities, and the planet. Though the work can seem daunting, nurses have an opportunity to imagine the futures we want to and to establish and grow communities of practice that can support us to equitably and ethically realize those goals. While numerous nurses are already innovating the creation and implementation of A.I. technologies, others are providing critical leadership in the realm of digital defense and refusal of unethical and weaponized forms of this tech. Nursing cannot afford to ignore widespread and growing abuses of A.I. tools and A.I.-enabled surveillance by state, industry and individual actors. Environmental and human costs of maintaining the infrastructure necessary for operation and widespread use of more resource-intensive forms of A.I. are currently unsustainable and therefore, unethical. It's also important to address ongoing challenges related to data quality, algorithmic bias, patient privacy, and consent to deliver safer and more equitable care for everyone. As nurses work towards greater health justice, we must be ready to integrate technologies and practices that move us closer to this goal, and to refuse and challenge those that do not. Table 6.4 summarizes additional resources for those who may wish to learn more about these important issues. We have also provided a series of case studies and reflection questions to prompt further discussions about A.I. and provision of safe, sustainable, and ethical nursing care.

Table 6.4 Additional resources

Category	Resource	Description
Health justice	Multifaceted approach for ethical and equitable implementation of artificial intelligence (AI) in public health and medicine Algorithmic justice league https://www.ajl.org/ Tech won't save us https://techwontsave.us/	Model designed to promote ethical and equitable implementation of A.I. Non-profit organization founded by A.I. researcher and "poet of code" joy Buolamwini, and focused on preventing and addressing algorithmic harms Podcast featuring leaders in A.I. and design justice
Consentful tech	Consentful tech project https://www.consentfultech.io	Website and zine supporting education in the design of more consentful tech
Patient safety	AI in healthcare safety hub (AHRQ): psnet.ahrq.gov/ai Coalition for Health A.I.: https://www.chai.org	Database of clinical incidents related to A.I., with learning modules Multidisciplinary working groups including nurses producing guidance for responsible A.I., A.I. model cards, registry, and other resources

Auditing A.I. Models and Clinical algorithms	REFORMS checklist https://reforms.cs.princeton.edu/#:~:text=The%20REFORMS%20checklist%20consists%20 of,social%20sciences%2C%20and%20health%20research. Algorithmic bias playbook https://www.ftc.gov/system/files/documents/public_events/1582978/algorithmic-bias-playbook.pdf	Reporting standards for machine learning-based science, designed to increase transparency and address A.I.-washing Publicly available guide to auditing clinical algorithms presented before the Federal Trade Commission [24]
Cybersecurity and digital defense	Care workers' digital defense toolkit https://nursingmutualaid.squarespace.com/defense Digital defense playbook (our data bodies project): www.odb.org Electronic frontier foundation surveillance self-defense toolkit https://ssd.eff.org	Nurse-centered toolkit summarizing individual and collective strategies care workers can use to defend against A.I.-related harms [23] Open-access workbook in English and Spanish, designed to facilitate discussions about surveillance and community defense Step-by-step guide and resources for safeguarding personal data security and privacy, including free software to reduce online tracking

(continued)

Table 6.4 (continued)

Category	Resource	Description
Occupational safety, whistleblowing and labor rights	Nurses' and patient's bill of rights: Guiding principles for A.I. Justice in nursing and health care http://bit.ly/4lGoTi2 Federal Labor Laws and the Department of Labor (https://www.dol.gov/agencies/whd/workers) Including protections for whistleblowers: https://www.dol.gov/general/topics/whistleblower Information about state-level whistleblower protections for health care workers from National Nurses United: https://www.nationalnursesunited.org/whistleblower-protection-laws-for-healthcare-workers	Statement of principles for A.I. justice developed by National Nurses United (NNU) Information about federal and state labor protections
Sustainability and planetary health	Alliance of nurses for healthy environments educational website: https://learning.envirn.org Anatomy of an A.I. System https://anatomyof.ai Low tech magazine https://solar.lowtechmagazine.com/about/what-is-low-tech-magazine/	Free, open-access educational materials, workshops, webinars and self-paced short courses from the Alliance of nurses for healthy environments (ANHE) Visual essay by Kate Crawford and Vladan Joler, depicting fractal chains of human and planetary resources required to manufacture a single smart speaker Solar-powered digital publication featuring examples of "low technology" designed to be sustainable

| Nursing education | The ethical use of artificial intelligence in nursing practice
https://www.nursingworld.org/globalassets/practiceandpolicy/nursing-excellence/ana-position-statements/the-ethical-use-of-artificial-intelligence-in-nursing-practice_bod-approved-12_20_22.pdf
Alternatives to Surveillant Technologies in Online Clinical Education
https://bit.ly/alternativesfornursinged
Artificial intelligence and academic professions
https://www.aaup.org/reports-publications/aaup-policies-reports/topical-reports/artificial-intelligence-and-academic | The American Nurses Association's official position statement on ethical use of A.I. in nursing care, published in 2022
An open-access resource guide developed by a large team of nurse educators from around the USA that outlines potential harms of some forms of A.I.-enabled ed. tech and possible alternatives
American Association of University Professors (AAUP) Task Force report on artificial intelligence and higher education, published in July 2025 |

6.12 End of Chapter Application Exercises

The following cases draw on real-life examples from lived experience, clinical, and community nursing practice. These scenarios are designed to provide opportunities for reflection, dialogue and application of knowledge from this chapter. We anticipate that as both the technology and contexts in which A.I. is applied continue to evolve, so will responses to these scenarios. There may be multiple valid responses to the accompanying reflection questions. Learners' perspectives are likely to vary based on their own positionality and experiences with A.I. For this reason, we have not provided definitive answer keys. We encourage readers to incorporate discussion of these cases as an active teaching and learning strategy.

6.12.1 Case 1: Ambient Intelligence for Documentation Support

A 68-year-old Haitian-American woman arrives at the emergency room after she fainted while gardening. She is accompanied by her adult daughter, who gave her a ride to the hospital. While sitting in the waiting room, the daughter notices a sign on the wall stating providers in the office use A.I. and ambient intelligence to assist with their documentation. When the triage nurse calls her mother back for her initial assessment, the adult daughter stops the nurse to express confusion and concern about what is being recorded. She wants to know who has access to the recordings, how they will be used, who has access, and how will this impact her mother's care?

Reflection Questions:
1. What are some of the potential benefits and risks of ambient intelligence when used for patient documentation in this scenario?
2. As the nurse, how might you approach the daughters' questions and patient education about ambient intelligence?
3. What nursing actions might support safe(r) and consentful use of ambient intelligence in this setting?
4. In your opinion, how does use of ambient intelligence like smart speakers and auto-scribes align with nursing considerations of health justice, sustainability, invisible labor, and digital defense?

6.12.2 Case 2: Continuous Remote Monitoring and Predictive Analytics

You are the nurse assigned to care for a patient with Type I diabetes in a home healthcare setting. The patient has just received a new wearable device that monitors their blood glucose levels and automatically adjusts their insulin pump to provide an appropriate dose. The proprietary device also pushes continuous monitoring data to a private company that uses software with A.I.-enabled predictive analytics. The software is designed to provide personalized recommendations for better glucose management. The patient can access this information and alerts via an app on their smartphone. During your visit, the patient expresses excitement to you that due to their new monitor, they will no longer have to pay close attention to their blood sugar levels.

Reflection Questions:
1. How might you respond to the patient's statement about no longer having to pay close attention to their blood glucose levels?
2. What might you recommend to the patient in terms of protecting their data privacy and digital defense?
3. The patient asks you for more information about their new monitor's predictive capabilities. Describe some of the considerations you would keep in mind when searching for and reviewing evidence of the predictive software's safety and performance? What might cause you to trust (or question) a particular report?

6.12.3 Case 3: Agentic A.I. and Nurse Advocacy

Your local community crisis center is considering using agentic A.I. from a private company to streamline their suicide prevention hotline. Proponents of the proposal argue research from the A.I. company shows that their tool is safe and will assist with continuity of care, reduce wait times, and provide additional resources for lower cost than hiring and training human staff. There have been heated city council meetings over this issue, specifically around residents' concerns about the plan and media reports about some forms of generative A.I. providing harmful responses, "hallucinating" incorrect information, or reinforcing psychosis. As a mental health nurse who has worked in this community for many years, you attend the public hearing to provide expert testimony.

Reflection Questions:
1. What aspects of the issue would you prioritize discussing during your limited time before the city council (often just 2–3 minutes)?
2. What would you keep in mind when evaluating evidence regarding the safety, efficacy, acceptability and sustainability of such a plan?
3. What recommendations, if any, would you give to the city council regarding their proposal? Do you have any personal hopes or concerns regarding such a plan?

Acknowledgements and Conflicts of Interest   The authors would like to acknowledge the influence and support of mentors and accountability partners Drs. Monica R. McLemore, Wanda Montalvo, Anna Valdez, and members of the Nursing Mutual Aid collective. This writing would not be possible without the community of practice at the University of Massachusetts Amherst, including fellow Health Tech for the People (HT4P) co-founders Drs. Ravi Karkar and Jess Dillard-Wright.

We have no conflicts of interest to report.

Author Statements *Rachel (Rae) Walker* (they/them) is a Professor, PhD Program Director, and the first nurse to be named an AAAS Invention Ambassador. Drawing on over 20 years of health care experience spanning 3 continents, they've led teams that have developed A.I. tools and technologies designed to address a wide variety of health challenges. Their privilege and positionality as a white queer and trans person informs their commitments to design justice, community-directed health innovation, and digital defense. They co-founded the Nursing Mutual Aid collective and Health Tech for the People, a transdisciplinary collaborative focused on A.I. design and tech ethics. They've consulted on national tech policy for organizations like Facebook and UnitedHealth, U.S. Patent and Trademark Office, White House Office of Science and Technology Policy and U.S. Department of Health and Human Services. They believe nursing care (including nursing education) is a dynamic, holistic and relational process that requires human imagination and creativity, co-creation, and consent.

Seyyedehmahdiyeh Khastar (she/her) is a nursing PhD student at the University of Massachusetts Amherst. Her research explores outcomes of agentic A.I. use in health care among persons who do not speak English and those with Low English Proficiency (LEP). She contributed to this chapter by synthesizing knowledge related to A.I.-related consent practices and diagnostics.

Francis Kuehnle (they/them) is a psychiatric nurse and educator with expertise in therapeutic communication and teaching through stories. Their position on AI is that they are tired of grading essays written by robots. Drawing on their clinical experience in acute care and community settings, they helped to craft case studies and reflections associated with this chapter.

Miaomiao Shen (she/her) is a PhD student in Nursing at the University of Massachusetts Amherst. Her research explores the integration of mHealth and A.I. technologies to support older adults, with a focus on cultural competence and health equity. She contributed to this chapter by synthesizing the evidence on predictive analytics applications in clinical nursing—examining ethical and practical implications for nursing practice.

Author's Note [RW]: As of the writing of this chapter, U.S. policy regarding A.I. development, deployment, and regulation continues to shift rapidly. Prior federal A.I. policy roadmaps like the White House Office of Science and Technology Policy's Blueprint for an A.I. Bill of Rights were rescinded by executive order in January 2025. Regulatory agencies with important roles in protecting public health and regulating health technologies like the U.S. Food and Drug Administration (FDA), Centers for Disease Control and Prevention (CDC), and Environmental Protection Agency (EPA) have undergone severe workforce reductions. The National Institute of Nursing Research (NINR) has also been eliminated. Numerous keywords associated with diversity, equity, inclusion and anti-racism have been scrubbed from websites, grants, and datasets—shaping outputs of any A.I. trained on them in the future. Sensitive government datasets that are typically kept siloed from each other—like social security information, Medicare and Medicaid records, and tax data—have been accessed by the recently-established Department of

Government Efficiency (DOGE) to train new A.I. tools designed to replace human workers. These datasets have also been used to assist the Department of Homeland Security in targeting specific groups for incarceration or deportation, such as immigrants. The full impacts of these changes are difficult to predict, but have already had significant effects on privacy, civil rights, population health and public trust.

References

1. American Association of Colleges of Nursing. The Essentials: Core competencies for professional nursing education. [Internet]. 2021 [cited 2025 Mar 20]. Available from: https://www.aacnnursing.org/essentials
2. Crawford K. Atlas of AI: power, politics, and the planetary costs of artificial intelligence. New Haven: Yale University Press; 2021. p. 336.
3. Narayanan A, Kapoor S. A.I. Snake oil: what artificial intelligence can do, what it can't, and how to tell the difference. Princeton University Press; 2024.
4. Katz Y. Artificial whiteness: politics and ideology in artificial intelligence. Columbia University Press; 2020.
5. McGrow K. Artificial intelligence: essentials for nursing. Nursing (Lond). 2019;49(9):46–9.
6. Costanza-Chock S. Design justice [Internet]. MIT Press; 2020 [cited 2024 Nov 8]. Available from: https://mitpress.mit.edu/9780262043458/design-justice/
7. Alang S, Blackstock O. Health justice: a framework for mitigating the impacts of HIV and COVID-19 on disproportionately affected communities. Am J Public Health [Internet]. 2023 Feb [cited 2024 Sept 21];113(2):194–201. Available from: https://ajph.aphapublications.org/doi/10.2105/AJPH.2022.307139
8. Bender EM, Hanna A. The A.I. Con: how to fight big tech's hype and create the future we want. HarperCollins; 2025.
9. Bazzano LA, Durant J, Brantley PR. A modern history of informed consent and the role of key information. Ochsner J [Internet]. 2021 [cited 2025 July 13];21(1):81–85. Available from: https://www.ncbi.nlm.nih.gov/pmc/articles/PMC7993430/
10. Amann J, Blasimme A, Vayena E, Frey D, Madai VI, Precise4Q Consortium. Explainability for artificial intelligence in healthcare: a multidisciplinary perspective. BMC Med Inform Decis Mak. 2020;20(1):310.
11. Penner SB, Mercado NR, Bernstein S, Erickson E, DuBois MA, Dreisbach C. Fostering informed consent and shared decision-making in maternity nursing with the advancement of artificial intelligence. MCN Am J Matern Child Nurs. 2025;50(2):78–85.
12. Chau M, Rahman MG, Debnath T. From black box to clarity: strategies for effective AI informed consent in healthcare. Artif Intell Med [Internet]. 2025 [cited 2025 July 17];167:103169. Available from: https://www.sciencedirect.com/science/article/pii/S0933365725001046
13. ANA Center for Ethics and Human Rights. The ethical use of artificial intelligence in nursing practice [Internet]. ANA; 2022. Available from: the-ethical-use-of-artificial-intelligence-in-nursing-practice_bod-approved-12_20_22.pdf.
14. Lee U, Tolliver D. Building Consentful tech [Internet]. Consentful Tech Project; 2017. Available from: https://www.consentfultech.io/
15. Alliance of Nurses for Healthy Environments. Nurses Climate Challenge [Internet]. [cited 2024 Nov 25]. Available from: https://envirn.org/nurses-climate-challenge/
16. Ueda D, Walston SL, Fujita S, Fushimi Y, Tsuboyama T, Kamagata K, et al. Climate change and artificial intelligence in healthcare: review and recommendations towards a sustainable future. Diagn Interv Imaging [Internet]. 2024 Nov 1 [cited 2025 July 14];105(11):453–459. Available from: https://www.sciencedirect.com/science/article/pii/S2211568424001384

17. Li P, Yang J, Islam MA, Ren S. Making AI less "thirsty": uncovering and addressing the secret water footprint of AI models [Internet]. arXiv; 2023 [cited 2025 July 13]. Available from: https://arxiv.org/abs/2304.03271

18. Crawford K. Generative AI's environmental costs are soaring — and mostly secret. Nature [Internet]. 2024 [cited 2025 Feb 20];626(8000):693–693. Available from: https://www.nature.com/articles/d41586-024-00478-x

19. Ronquillo CE, Peltonen L, Pruinelli L, Chu CH, Bakken S, Beduschi A, et al. Artificial intelligence in nursing: priorities and opportunities from an international invitational think-tank of the nursing and artificial intelligence leadership collaborative. J Adv Nurs John Wiley Sons Inc. 2021;77(9):3707–17.

20. Pavuluri S, Sangal R, Sather J, Taylor RA. Balancing act: the complex role of artificial intelligence in addressing burnout and healthcare workforce dynamics. BMJ Health Care Inform [Internet]. 2024 [cited 2025 July 13];31(1):e101120. Available from: https://informatics.bmj.com/lookup/doi/10.1136/bmjhci-2024-101120

21. Elish MC, Watkins EA. Data & society. Data & Society Research Institute; 2020. [cited 2025 Feb 13]. Repairing Innovation. Available from: https://datasociety.net/library/repairing-innovation/

22. $9 AI "nurses"? Inside the NVIDIA-Hippocratic AI collaboration [Internet]. MedTech Pulse. 2024. [cited 2025 Feb 15]. Available from: https://www.medtechpulse.com/article/insight/ai-nurses

23. Walker R. Digital defense toolkit: protecting ourselves from artificial intelligence-related harms. Online J Issues Nurs. 2025;30(2)

24. Obermeyer Z, Powers B, Vogeli C, Mullainathan S. Dissecting racial bias in an algorithm used to manage the health of populations. Science [Internet]. 2019 [cited 2025 Feb 20];366(6464):447–453. Available from: https://www.science.org/doi/10.1126/science.aax2342

25. Benjamin R. Race after technology: abolitionist tools for the new Jim code [Internet]. Polity; 2020 [cited 2024 Nov 22]. Available from: https://www.wiley.com/en-nl/Race+After+Technology%3A+Abolitionist+Tools+for+the+New+Jim+Code-p-9781509526437

26. Dillard-Wright J, Shields-Haas V. Nursing with the people: reimagining futures for nursing. ANS Adv Nurs Sci. 2021;44(3):195–209.

27. ANA [Internet]. 2022 [cited 2025 May 30]. Commission's foundational report on racism in nursing. Available from: https://www.nursingworld.org/practice-policy/workforce/racism-in-nursing/national-commission-to-address-racism-in-nursing/commissions-foundational-report-on-racism%2D%2Din-nursing/

28. Roy B, Riley C, Sears L, Rula EY. Collective well-being to improve population health outcomes: an actionable conceptual model and review of the literature. Am J Health Promot [Internet]. 2018 Nov [cited 2025 Feb 9];32(8):1800–13. Available from: http://silk.library.umass.edu/login?url=https://search.ebscohost.com/login.aspx?direct=true&db=s3h&AN=132632907&site=ehost-live&scope=site

29. Eubanks V. Automating inequality: how high-tech tools profile, police and punish the poor [Internet]. St. Martin's Press; 2018 [cited 2025 July 16]. Available from: https://us.macmillan.com/books/9781250074317/automatinginequality/

30. Walker A. Nurse.org. [cited 2025 July 17]. Bill banning AI from using the title "nurse" is approved in OR—only humans are nurses. Available from:. https://nurse.org/news/nurse-ai-ban-law/

31. Olson P. Forbes. [cited 2025 July 18]. Nearly half of all 'AI startups' are cashing in on hype. Available from: https://www.forbes.com/sites/parmyolson/2019/03/04/nearly-half-of-all-ai-startups-are-cashing-in-on-hype/

32. Mitchell M, Wu S, Zaldivar A, Barnes P, Vasserman L, Hutchinson B, et al. Model cards for model reporting. In: Proceedings of the Conference on Fairness, Accountability, and Transparency [Internet]. 2019 [cited 2025 Mar 18]. p. 220–229. Available from: http://arxiv.org/abs/1810.03993

33. Fagherazzi G, Fischer A, Ismael M, Despotovic V. Voice for health: the use of vocal bio-markers from research to clinical practice. Digit Biomark [Internet]. 2021 [cited 2025 July 18];5(1):78–88. Available from: https://www.ncbi.nlm.nih.gov/pmc/articles/PMC8138221/

34. Kathleen. FDA approves first AI-powered skin cancer Diagnostic tool [Internet]. AIM at Melanoma Foundation 2024 [cited 2025 July 18]. Available from: https://www.aimatmela-noma.org/ai-powered-diagnostics/

35. Campo-Prieto P, Cancela-Carral JM, Rodríguez-Fuentes G. Wearable immersive vir-tual reality device for promoting physical activity in Parkinson's disease patients. Sensors (Basel) [Internet]. 2022 [cited 2025 July 18];22(9):3302. Available from: https://www.mdpi.com/1424-8220/22/9/3302

36. Levine A. Suicide hotline shares data with for-profit spinoff, raising ethical questions. POLITICO [Internet] 2022 [cited 2025 July 18]; Available from: https://www.politico.com/news/2022/01/28/suicide-hotline-silicon-valley-privacy-debates-00002617

37. Greaves J, Colucci E. Crisis-line workers' perspectives on AI in suicide prevention: a qualita-tive exploration of risk and opportunity BMC Public Health [Internet]. 2025 [cited 2025 July 18];25(1):2229. Available from: https://doi.org/10.1186/s12889-025-23298-8

38. Shachar C, Killelea A, Gerke S. AI and health insurance prior authorization: regulators need to step up oversight. [cited 2025 July 18]; Available from: https://www.healthaffairs.org/do/10.1377/forefront.20240703.824037/full/

39. Sutton RT, Pincock D, Baumgart DC, Sadowski DC, Fedorak RN, Kroeker KI. An overview of clinical decision support systems: benefits, risks, and strategies for success. NPJ Digit Med [Internet]. 2020 Feb 6 [cited 2025 Mar 18];3(1):1–10. Available from: https://www.nature.com/articles/s41746-020-0221-y

40. Lee HP, Sarkar A, Tankelevitch L, Drosos I, Rintel S, Banks R, et al. The impact of generative AI on critical thinking: self-reported reductions in cognitive effort and confidence effects from a survey of knowledge workers. CHI Conf Hum Factors Comput Syst CHI '25 April 26–May 01 2025 Yokohama Jpn ACM N Y NY USA 2025.

41. Goh E, Gallo R, Hom J, Strong E, Weng Y, Kerman H, et al. Large language model influ-ence on diagnostic reasoning: a randomized clinical trial. JAMA Netw Open [Internet]. 2024 Oct 28 [cited 2025 July 28];7(10):e2440969. Available from: https://doi.org/10.1001/jamanetworkopen.2024.40969

42. Keim-Malpass J, Moorman LP. Nursing and precision predictive analytics monitoring in the acute and intensive care setting: an emerging role for responding to COVID-19 and beyond. Int J Nurs Stud Adv [Internet]. 2021 Nov 1 [cited 2025 July 17];3:100019. Available from: https://www.sciencedirect.com/science/article/pii/S2666142X21000011

43. Rossetti SC, Dykes PC, Knaplund C, Cho S, Withall J, Lowenthal G, et al. Real-time surveil-lance system for patient deterioration: a pragmatic cluster-randomized controlled trial. Nat Med [Internet] 2025 June [cited 2025 July 17];31(6):1895–1902. Available from: https://www.nature.com/articles/s41591-025-03609-7

44. National Nurses United. Nurses and patients bill of rights: guiding principles for A.I. justice in nursing and health care [Internet]. Available from: https://www.nationalnursesunited.org/sites/default/files/nnu/documents/0424_NursesPatients-BillOfRights_Principles-AI-Justice_flyer.pdf

45. Brydges G. Artificial intelligence in nursing practice: decisional support, clinical integration, and future directions. OJIN Online J Issues Nurs [Internet] 2025 [cited 2025 July 17];30(2). Available from: https://ojin.nursingworld.org/table-of-contents/volume-30-2025/number-2-may-2025/artificial-intelligence-in-nursing-practice-decisional-support-clinical-integra-tion-and-future-directions/

46. Application of Artificial Intelligence in Symptom Monitoring in Adult Cancer Survivorship: A Systematic Review | JCO Clinical Cancer Informatics [Internet]. [cited 2025 July 28]. Available from: https://ascopubs.org/doi/10.1200/CCI.24.00119

47. van de Sande D, van Genderen ME, Verhoef C, Huiskens J, Gommers D, van Unen E, et al. Optimizing discharge after major surgery using an artificial intelligence–based decision sup-port tool (DESIRE): an external validation study. Surgery [Internet] 2022 [cited 2025 July

28];172(2):663–669. Available from: https://www.sciencedirect.com/science/article/pii/S003960602200215X

48. Patel H, Hassell A, Keniston A, Davis C. Impact of remote patient monitoring on length of stay for patients with COVID-19. Telemed J E-Health Off J Am Telemed Assoc. 2023;29(2):298–303.

49. Phelan SM, Burkhartzmeyer HL, Standen EC, Arcand LL, Kiker KM, Simiele KC, et al. A virtual reality intervention to increase interracial empathy and upstander behaviors in nursing leaders. Soc Sci Med [Internet]. 2025 [cited 2025 Aug 5];366:117648. Available from: https://www.sciencedirect.com/science/article/pii/S027795362401102X

50. Șerban O, Thapen N, Maginnis B, Hankin C, Foot V. Real-time processing of social media with SENTINEL: a syndromic surveillance system incorporating deep learning for health classification. Inf Process Manag [Internet]. 2019 [cited 2025 July 14];56(3):1166–84. Available from: https://www.sciencedirect.com/science/article/pii/S0306457317303448

51. Andersen ES, Birk-Korch JB, Hansen RS, Fly LH, Röttger R, Arcani DMC, et al. Monitoring performance of clinical artificial intelligence in health care: a scoping review. JBI Evid Synth. 2024;22(12):2423–46.

52. Rockenschaub P, Akay EM, Carlisle BG, Hilbert A, Wendland J, Meyer-Eschenbach F, et al. External validation of AI-based scoring systems in the ICU: a systematic review and meta-analysis. BMC Med Inform Decis Mak [Internet]. 2025 [cited 2025 July 17];25(1):1–10. Available from: https://research.ebsco.com/linkprocessor/plink?id=953eb291-71d2-36ec-84fe-4d4ce3f555d2

53. Alderden J, Kennerly SM, Wilson A, Dimas J, McFarland C, Yap DY, et al. Explainable artificial intelligence for predicting hospital-acquired pressure injuries in COVID-19–positive critical care patients. Comput Inform Nurs [Internet] 2022 [cited 2025 July 18];40(10):659–665. Available from: https://www.ncbi.nlm.nih.gov/pmc/articles/PMC9555852/

54. Hasan N, Ahmed MF. Wearable technology for elderly care: integrating health monitoring and emergency alerts. J Comput Netw Commun [Internet]. 2024 [cited 2025 Feb 20];2024(1):5593708. Available from: https://onlinelibrary.wiley.com/doi/abs/10.1155/jcnc/5593708

55. Liu S, Wright AP, McCoy AB, Huang SS, Steitz B, Wright A. Detecting emergencies in patient portal messages using large language models and knowledge graph-based retrieval-augmented generation. J Am Med Inform Assoc JAMIA [Internet]. 2025 [cited 2025 July 28];32(6):1032–1039. Available from: https://www.ncbi.nlm.nih.gov/pmc/articles/PMC12089757/

56. Dillard-Wright J. Electronic health record as a panopticon: a disciplinary apparatus in nursing practice. Nurs Philos. 2019;20(2):e12239.

57. Wells KJ, Spilda FU. Uber for nursing: how an AI-powered gig model is threatening health care [Internet]. The Roosevelt Institute; 2024 Dec [cited 2025 Feb 15]. Available from: https://rooseveltinstitute.org/publications/uber-for-nursing/

Kellie Bryant, Michael J. Jabbour,
and Delaney Wright La Rosa

Definition of Keywords

Artificial Intelligence (AI): The simulation of human intelligence in machines, especially in tasks like pattern recognition, decision-making, and natural language processing. In nursing, AI is used for clinical decision support, documentation, and education.

Large Language Models (LLMs): A type of AI trained on massive datasets to generate human-like text. Examples include ChatGPT and GPT-4, which can draft clinical notes, simulate conversations, or support student learning.

Predictive Algorithms: Tools that use data to forecast outcomes, such as early detection of sepsis or patient deterioration. In nursing education, they demonstrate real-world AI applications.

Adaptive Simulations: Learning environments that change based on a student's responses, powered by AI to mimic real-life clinical variation and complexity.

AI Literacy: The ability to understand, critically assess, and effectively use AI tools. For nurse educators and students, this includes ethical, technical, and practical knowledge.

Automation Bias: The tendency to over-rely on AI outputs or automated systems, which can lead to missed errors or poor clinical judgment.

K. Bryant (✉)
Center for Innovation in Education Excellence, National League for Nursing,
Washington, DC, USA
e-mail: kbryant@nln.org

M. J. Jabbour
Office of CTO, Microsoft, New York City, NY, USA
e-mail: michael.jabbour@gmail.com

D. W. La Rosa
Florida State University College of Nursing, Tallahassee, FL, USA
e-mail: DWLaRosa@fsu.edu

D. W. La Rosa et al. (eds.), *Nursing Education in the AI Era*,
https://doi.org/10.1007/978-3-032-12402-9_7

Futures Thinking (Strategic Foresight): A structured approach to anticipating and preparing for long-term change, used to align nursing education with emerging healthcare and technological trends.

Horizon Scanning: The process of identifying early signals of change, such as new technologies or social shifts, that may impact the future of nursing practice and education.

7.1   Introduction and Overview

Artificial intelligence has slipped from healthcare's periphery into its beating heart. It is no longer simply a technology to be implemented but a vital sign that educators, practitioners, and students alike must learn to read. From wartime logic machines to today's generative systems that draft clinical guidelines as fluently as they analyze radiographs, AI's evolution has created both opportunity and urgency for nurses. As the traditional quarterbacks of multidisciplinary care, nurses now operate in environments where predictive algorithms catch sepsis hours before traditional clinical signs appear, where voice-first documentation returns nurses to bedside care, and where adaptive simulations build complex thinking that once took years of bedside practice.

These innovations bring profound questions. Issues of privacy, bias, and the human touch that defines nursing practice cannot be overlooked. Building AI literacy requires more than technical training; it demands reflection on what it means to care, advocate, and decide in an environment increasingly mediated by data. Regulatory frameworks are not obstacles but essential guardrails, ensuring that technology augments rather than replaces what is irreplaceable: human judgment, compassion, and presence. The narrative thread of nursing remains intact. When humans stay at the center and in the loop, AI shifts from a bewildering black box to a trusted teammate, surfacing patterns before they become problems. This is not about replacing nursing intelligence. It is about creating opportunities for nurses to make better decisions while deepening, rather than diminishing, the human connection at healthcare's heart.

Across classrooms, clinics, and communities worldwide, educators are challenged to anticipate these shifts. They must prepare graduates not only for today's realities but for dynamic systems of care that demand both technological fluency and enduring relational skill. Anticipating these changes through intentional educational design will be critical to sustaining nursing's impact in a rapidly evolving healthcare landscape.

7.2   Evolution of AI: From Historical Curiosity to Clinical Core

Artificial intelligence did not emerge overnight. Its evolution can be understood through two broad eras that trace the journey from distant curiosity to essential partner in healthcare. The first era stretched from roughly the 1940s through the early 2000s [1]. During this time, neural networks began to take shape while Alan Turing decrypted wartime codes. Psychiatry labs experimented with conversational programs like ELIZA, while engineers worked to extract clean ECG signals from noisy recordings [2–5]. Although fascinating, these advances remained largely invisible to practicing nurses who continued to chart by hand and calculate medication dosages manually. For most clinicians, AI was something confined to research papers or science fiction.

The second era, beginning around 2011, brought AI directly into healthcare's operational core [6]. IBM's Watson consumed millions of pages of medical literature and famously defeated human champions on Jeopardy, sparking widespread attention beyond computer science circles. Deep learning models rapidly outpaced earlier systems in recognizing complex patterns, setting new standards in fields like radiology. By 2020, large language models such as GPT-3 demonstrated the capacity to generate coherent, contextually aware narratives that could approximate human-written clinical notes [7, 8]. Today, surveys indicate that approximately 80 percent of healthcare organizations worldwide report using at least one AI application. These systems are now part of daily workflows and shape decisions that impact patient outcomes.

For nursing, these shifts are not just milestones in computer science. They reveal how AI has moved from the background to become a silent collaborator in the patient care environment [9]. Predictive algorithms can flag early signs of sepsis, prompting interventions well before traditional vital signs change. Voice documentation tools allow nurses to narrate assessments in real time, reducing time spent away from patients. Adaptive simulations adjust based on learner decisions, building subtle layers of clinical judgment that were once possible only through repeated bedside exposure over many years. Each of these examples underscores why nursing education must engage fully with this evolving landscape.

This trajectory is also a signal to educators that AI is more than a set of technical innovations. Around the world, organizations such as the World Health Organization, UNESCO, and the World Economic Forum have recognized that emerging technologies like AI represent structural changes. These shifts are expected to reconfigure how labor, health systems, and global care coordination operate [10, 11]. They use tools like horizon scanning and strategic foresight to identify early signals, plan for complex scenarios, and shape future systems rather than merely react. Nursing education stands at a similar threshold. By recognizing how AI has moved from early theoretical experiments to deeply embedded systems, educators can plan more deliberately. This means designing curricula and faculty development programs that prepare graduates to work in care environments where AI is not an accessory but a foundational element. It also means teaching students to question data outputs, to recognize when a predictive model might miss critical cultural or contextual factors, and to advocate for patients when technology's conclusions need to be tempered by human insight. Preparing for this future means looking beyond immediate tool adoption toward long-range strategies that sustain nursing's ethical commitments within a rapidly changing world.

7.3   Preparing Students for Evolving Practice

In American football, the quarterback reads the defense, calls the audible, and distributes the ball. In clinical reality, the nurses do the same. Nurses triage alarms, brief physicians, cue pharmacy, calm families, and coordinate the entire care team. This quarterback metaphor comes alive when we witness AI removing clipboard chores so nurses can focus on the plays that matter most.

Consider early-warning algorithms that flag sepsis or hemorrhage hours before manual detection, transforming a desperate scramble into a planned intervention. Imagine voice-driven charting systems that have reduced keyboard time by a third. Nurses describe the feeling as mentally returning to the bedside rather than remaining tethered to screens. Picture simulation centers where AI-driven patients respond to student actions with evolving vital signs and dialogue, creating learning environments that adapt to each future nurse's decisions. These are not mere conveniences. They are new muscle memory, requiring retraining of clinical reflexes. When nurses can trust these next-play suggestions, they gain precious seconds that often determine not just vital signs, but entire family futures.

Recent conversations with nursing leaders across the country revealed deeply human concerns. A generational divide has formed. Sixty percent of staff are Gen Z, digital natives comfortable with smartphones but not necessarily AI-fluent. Meanwhile, veteran colleagues worry about being replaced by a typo. Both groups need different pathways toward competence and confidence [12, 13].

There is also profound fatigue with traditional training approaches. Another mandatory module feels like spam in an already cluttered clinical inbox. Leaders are seeking a more organic approach, inspiration that sparks curiosity, plain-language demystification that builds confidence, and hands-on practice with real nursing use-cases. This mirrors what Nightingale knew intuitively. Change sticks when it is peer-taught, outcome-visible, and centered on patient wellbeing.

AI-powered personalization is poised to reshape nursing education by aligning instructional design with the unique strengths, needs, and pacing of each learner [1–3]. Rather than advancing all students through a uniform sequence of lectures and exams, emerging systems will dynamically assess performance, adapt content delivery, and optimize timing for reinforcement or remediation. Competency-based education, once largely time-bound and paper-based, will evolve into responsive, data-rich environments where students receive curated learning paths informed by their real-time progress.

Learning analytics generated through student interactions with virtual simulations, quizzes, discussion forums, and clinical case tools will be synthesized by AI systems to identify areas of conceptual weakness [2, 4, 5]. These systems can also flag patterns of disengagement and suggest targeted resources or faculty outreach. The learning management system will become not just a repository, but a predictive engine. While this holds promise for addressing equity gaps through individualized support, it also requires a major reconfiguration of faculty roles, curriculum design, and feedback structures.

This transformation means that new nurses may graduate with individualized skill profiles shaped by precision learning. Preceptors and clinical employers may encounter graduates who are exceptionally prepared in some areas but require focused support in others. This could lead to more efficient onboarding and tailored career development, especially if employers have access to AI-enhanced skills transcripts that detail competencies and learning preferences. However, it may also challenge traditional orientation models that assume a uniform baseline, emphasizing the need for collaborative dialogue between educational institutions and practice sites to align expectations and support new graduates effectively.

> **Quarterbacking Under Pressure: Reading AI's Signal When Every Second Counts**
> The hallway lights dim after midnight, but the vigilance never fades. A charge nurse glances between six telemetry screens, her eyes catching subtle patterns. A new graduate recalculates an insulin dose, triple-checking her math. A night-shift veteran studies Room 214's lab trends, wondering why potassium keeps dropping despite replacement. Across thousands of hospitals, these quiet heroes share an unspoken wish: "Give me the signal before the crisis hits."

7.4   Transforming Educator Roles

Technology courses once nestled safely in "informatics electives." That era has ended. AI literacy now represents a core safety competency comparable to medication mathematics or sterile technique. Faculty champions can create learning pathways that pair clinical pain-points with safe AI experiments, using large language models to draft teaching materials, validating them for readability and bias, or employing a predictive tool to draft teaching materials and then validating them for readability and bias. They might also employ predictive tools to identify high-risk patients and discuss cases where the algorithm could miss subtle clinical signs. These iterative experiences build institutional comfort more effectively than top-down mandates or theoretical lectures.

At its heart, this transformation is not about replacing human judgment but augmenting it [6]. Machines compress latency, but humans confer meaning. An AI system may generate multiple care plans in seconds, yet it is often the nurse who notices when a patient's whispered fears or a scribbled note on a napkin changes the trajectory of care. True agency arises from lived experience, not silicon circuits.

The boundary between human and machine intelligence highlights that algorithms operate in "small worlds" of well-defined problems, while nurses practice in "large worlds" filled with ambiguity. Each AI implementation must ensure there is enough context for compassionate judgment and enough space for asking why, not just answering what.

As AI reshapes the landscape of nursing education and clinical environments, the role of the nurse educator must also expand. Faculty will increasingly serve as data interpreters, helping students make sense of AI-generated insights, question automated outputs, and identify when technology must yield to human ethics or intuition. In this way, educators become guides not just through course content, but through the larger epistemology of how knowledge is created, evaluated, and applied.

Educators will also function as ethical stewards, ensuring that AI tools used in the classroom or clinical lab are transparent, inclusive, and aligned with culturally responsive care. They will be called to partner with IT leaders and instructional designers, contributing nursing expertise to the selection, customization, and oversight of AI platforms. This collaborative leadership is essential to avoid defaulting to technologies built solely on engineering priorities, which may miss critical nuances in patient experience or equity.

At the same time, preceptors in practice settings will face similar challenges. As students arrive with experience using AI-powered simulations, documentation tools, and predictive dashboards, clinical mentors will need to help them apply these systems with clinical nuance. They may also find themselves navigating care environments where AI recommendations are deeply embedded, requiring a balanced supervision style that supports learning while reinforcing independent clinical judgment.

This evolution means that traditional boundaries between academic educators and clinical preceptors will become more porous. Faculty and preceptors may jointly monitor student progression through shared AI dashboards or coordinate feedback across settings. These integrated roles will demand new communication systems and shared accountability structures. Ultimately, nurse educators and clinical mentors together will model how to lead, critique, and care within complex technological ecosystems, ensuring that nursing's moral center is not lost amid automation.

7.5   Risks, Bias, and Ethical Stewardship

Regulators worldwide are crafting guardrails that address these concerns. The EU AI Act categorizes most clinical AI as "high-risk," requiring transparency and human oversight [7]. FDA principles demand ongoing monitoring and clinician-in-the-loop design [8]. The World Health Organization has established ethical pillars from autonomy to sustainability [9]. Together, these frameworks are not intended to constrain innovation but to channel it like riverbanks guiding water toward productive rather than destructive ends.

The challenge of equity deserves special attention. AI's promise of personalized medicine collapses if algorithms carry structural biases. A sobering study revealed an algorithm underestimating illness severity for Black patients by 25 percent, not from malicious design but because it used historical healthcare spending rather than physiological markers [10]. This finding reminds us that technology inherits societal blind spots unless we intentionally correct course.

For educators preparing tomorrow's nurses, this means conducting curricular equity audits to ensure case libraries include diverse phenotypes, accents, and family structures. It means teaching students to question who is missing from training data, extending culturally congruent care into the digital domain. Most importantly, it means maintaining human judgment as the final arbiter when algorithmic outputs conflict with lived experience or patient narratives.

As the healthcare landscape continues to evolve, nurse educators must be equipped to revise and adapt existing curricula to prepare future nurses for practice in increasingly AI-integrated environments. A critical first step is building a strong foundation in AI and developing AI literacy among nurse educators. Similar to the adoption curve of other emerging technologies, resistance to AI implementation is common and often stems from a lack of knowledge or familiarity with these tools. In a 2024 survey conducted by the American Nurses Association involving 7200 nurses, 36 percent reported not understanding how to use AI [11]. This gap can significantly contribute to hesitation around adoption, underscoring the need for clear guidelines, resources, and training to support faculty in integrating AI into their teaching practices.

Equally important to demonstrating utility is addressing the potential risks and ethical considerations of AI in education. Concerns related to academic integrity, AI-induced automation bias, and diminished critical thinking must be acknowledged and proactively addressed. Assignments that require students to critically evaluate AI-generated outputs, such as patient education materials or clinical recommendations, can help promote responsible AI use while reinforcing clinical judgment. These approaches are especially important as traditional assessment methods, like multiple-choice exams and essays, become increasingly vulnerable to automation.

As AI integration accelerates, attention must be paid to issues of access and equity. The financial and infrastructural demands associated with AI adoption may disproportionately affect under-resourced institutions and underserved student populations. It is imperative that access to AI tools and education is democratized to avoid exacerbating existing disparities. Ensuring equitable access to AI technologies is essential not only for educational equity but also for addressing global healthcare challenges and mitigating the ongoing nursing workforce shortage.

The future of AI in nursing education will not be shaped solely by whether these technologies are adopted, but by how thoughtfully they are integrated and governed. This means educators and institutions must engage deeply with issues of data justice, regulatory alignment, and patient safety. Shared governance with accreditation bodies and licensing agencies will be critical to ensure that AI-enhanced teaching and assessment methods meet rigorous standards and do not inadvertently entrench biases.

Students must also learn to interrogate algorithmic outputs, understand the limitations of predictive models, and appreciate where human intuition, cultural knowledge, or ethical reasoning rightly override automated suggestions. By fostering critical engagement with AI rather than passive reliance, nurse educators can prepare graduates who not only use these tools competently but also steward them responsibly. In doing so, the profession can ensure that AI becomes a force for expanding equity and compassion in healthcare rather than narrowing its scope.

> *Fast forward to a nightshift in the near future: It's 3:17 AM. Room 214 triggers an alarm.* The predictive dashboard quietly flashes: "Risk of septic shock in 6 hours." The bedside nurse glances, speaks a brief note that automatically populates the chart, and pages rapid response before vital signs visibly deteriorate. The team stabilizes the patient; the family never experiences the trauma of a code-blue sprint. Nobody applauds the algorithm. They recognize the nurse who read the defense and changed the play.

7.6 Equity, Inclusion, and Global Access

Addressing these challenges will require intentional planning and cross-sector collaboration. Programs must advocate for institutional investment in equitable access and consider open-source or low-bandwidth AI tools that can reach students regardless of geographic or economic barriers. Curriculum leaders should ensure all students receive explicit training in AI use, not just passive exposure, so fluency is not mistaken for privilege or vice versa. AI holds real potential to democratize education, but only if its implementation is deliberately designed to do so.

This is fundamentally a justice issue, not simply a matter of technical infrastructure. Ensuring inclusive AI integration means interrogating who benefits, who is left behind, and how we can build systems that truly support diverse learners and communities. In doing so, nurse educators can transform the promise of AI into a reality that closes gaps rather than widens them, creating pathways to advanced practice and leadership for all students, no matter where they begin.

7.7 Horizon Scanning and Futures Thinking

Artificial intelligence is advancing at a rate that outpaces most institutional processes, including those in nursing education. While the last few years have brought substantial attention to present-day applications, generative tools, decision support systems, and automated documentation, less attention has been paid to the horizon. These shifts in education cannot be separated from parallel transformations in clinical practice, public health infrastructure, and global care delivery. As AI reshapes the way nurses are trained, it simultaneously alters the environments into which they graduate, making alignment between educational design and practice realities more critical than ever.

What comes next? How do we prepare nurse educators and students for a future that is not only uncertain but also rapidly forming in real time? Most academic programs are not built for this pace of change. Even as nurse educators explore AI tools like ChatGPT or voice dictation software, these implementations often remain piecemeal, reactive, or locked in faculty development silos. Conversations tend to focus on whether AI is being used, not on how it is reshaping the context of learning itself. This present-centered focus is understandable and even necessary for immediate capacity-building, but it is insufficient. Nursing education must now make a turn toward intentional future readiness.

To do so requires more than speculation. It requires a structured way of thinking about the future. Futures thinking, also known as strategic foresight, is the discipline of identifying early signals, projecting long-range scenarios, and planning for multiple possible outcomes. It is the approach used by global organizations like the World Health Organization, UNESCO, and the World Economic Forum when preparing for societal shifts in health, technology, and labor [12]. At its core, futures thinking does not predict the future; it prepares educators and institutions to influence what unfolds.

A key concept in futures thinking is horizon scanning, the deliberate search for weak signals that may indicate emerging trends. These signals often appear at the margins. Experimental AI tutors, modular credentialing systems, adaptive assessment tools, or voice-based clinical training may seem peripheral today, but collectively, they shape the landscape nurse educators will soon inhabit. By paying attention to these developments early, educators can adapt curriculum, pedagogy, and policy in ways that ensure nursing remains a human-centered, equity-driven profession, rather than being reshaped by external forces.

The AACN Essentials offer an implicit endorsement of future-oriented curriculum [13]. Domains such as Data, Information, and Technology and Quality and Safety call for fluency in digital systems, adaptability to innovation, and critical engagement with technology. These competencies are not limited to the tools currently available. They anticipate a dynamic learning environment in which clinical reasoning, ethical practice, and data fluency must coexist.

Looking ahead, several weak signals are already emerging that will likely influence nursing education. Multimodal AI systems that process voice, image, video, and text in real time may enable advanced simulation and patient education. Autonomous AI agents that complete tasks without direct prompts could support course design or triage in clinical environments. Emotion recognition and engagement AI tools raise ethical concerns, but may also help monitor student wellbeing and burnout. Microcredentialing ecosystems, which stack skill-based digital credentials, may pressure programs to modularize outcomes and redefine global workforce pathways. While these trends begin in education, they do not end there. They signal a restructuring of the entire continuum from learning to practice.

By adopting horizon scanning and embedding futures thinking into faculty development and curriculum strategy, nurse educators can remain proactive. They will be better equipped to design programs that uphold equity, cultural humility, and relational care, even as technology transforms the structures around them. This is not simply about using AI; it is about preparing for the systems it will create and ensuring those systems reflect the core values of nursing.

7.8   Building Futures Literacy for Educators

As AI reshapes educational and clinical practice, building futures literacy among nurse educators becomes essential. Faculty must be supported not only in acquiring technical proficiency but in developing a mindset of critical foresight. This means creating space for reflective practice where educators can explore how their teaching identities, ethical commitments, and epistemological assumptions intersect with emerging technologies. Workshops and faculty learning communities can help make this work explicit, giving educators tools to anticipate and interrogate the societal impacts of AI.

Futures literacy also involves equipping educators to scan for early signals and prepare students for multiple potential scenarios. It demands that faculty model thoughtful skepticism, teaching students to question data provenance, algorithmic design, and whose interests are served by technological adoption. This is how students learn to navigate uncertainty with both confidence and humility.

Finally, as academic and clinical environments converge through shared dashboards, AI-supported onboarding, and cross-institutional learning systems, educators, and preceptors must collaborate more intentionally. Joint professional development sessions, co-designed case studies, and shared outcome reviews can help align expectations and foster a unified approach to guiding students. In doing so, nurse educators across settings can ensure that AI becomes a tool for expanding human care, not narrowing it.

7.9   Conclusion

Throughout this chapter, we have explored how AI can serve as a silent scout team while nurses remain trusted to call the audible, ensuring patient wellbeing remains at the center. With thoughtful integration, AI will amplify, not diminish, the human connection that defines nursing at its best. The integration of AI into nursing education offers both disruption and extraordinary possibility. Whether it becomes a source of fragmentation or a catalyst for flourishing depends on how educators, institutions, and regulatory bodies engage with these changes now. The future of nursing education will be defined not only by how skillfully we adopt new technologies, but by how intentionally we design systems that uphold relational care, cultural humility, and equity.

Faculty, students, and nurse leaders have an opportunity to guide this transformation thoughtfully. This is not about rejecting technology or surrendering to it. It is about embedding AI within a vision of nursing that keeps human connection and patient dignity at the center. The next chapter of nursing education will be written by those who have the courage to imagine it and the discipline to build it wisely.

The Future Play: Silent Scout Team
AI as the silent scout team, nurses as quarterbacks still trusted to call the audible, patients as the ones who win the game. The technology will continue evolving, but the core mission remains unchanged: to heal, to comfort, to advocate, to teach. With thoughtful integration, AI becomes not a replacement for these nursing arts but their amplifier, creating more space for the human connection that has always defined our profession at its best.

References

1. Ceruzzi P. A history of modern computing. 2nd ed. The MIT Press; 2003.
2. Jones LD, Golan D, Hanna SA, Ramachandran M. Artificial intelligence, machine learning and the evolution of healthcare: a bright future or cause for concern? Bone Jt Res. 2018;7(3):223–5.
3. Eldin S, Kaboudan A. Driven medical imaging platform: advancements in image analysis and healthcare diagnosis. Salah Eldin W Kaboudan 2023 AI-Driven Med Imaging Platf Adv Image Anal Healthc Diagn. J ACS Adv Comput Sci. 2023;14 https://doi.org/10.21608/asc.2024.248278.1018.
4. Muneer S, Ghazal TM, Alyas T, Raza MA, Abbas S, AlZoubi O, et al. Explainable AI-driven Chatbot system for heart disease prediction using machine learning. Int J Adv Comput Sci Appl [Internet] 2024 [cited 2025 Jun 29];15(12). Available from: http://thesai.org/Publications/View Paper?Volume=15&Issue=12&Code=ijacsa&SerialNo=27
5. Sun L, Liu D, Wang M, Han Y, Zhang Y, Zhou B, et al. Taming unleashed large language models with Blockchain for massive personalized reliable healthcare. IEEE J Biomed Health Inform. 2025;29(6):4498–511.
6. Chandrasekar R. Elementary? Question answering, IBM'S Watson, and the jeopardy! Challenge. Resonance. 2014;19(3):222–41.
7. Sezgin E, Sirrianni J, Linwood SL. Operationalizing and implementing Pretrained, large artificial intelligence linguistic models in the US health care system: outlook of generative Pretrained transformer 3 (GPT-3) as a service model. JMIR Med Inform. 2022;10(2):e32875.
8. Dehouche N. Plagiarism in the age of massive generative pre-trained transformers (GPT-3). Ethics Sci Environ Polit. 2021;21:17–23.
9. Shuaib A. Transforming healthcare with AI: promises, pitfalls, and pathways forward. Int J Gen Med. 2024;17:1765–71.
10. Sanin C. Artificial intelligence: current perspectives and alternative paths. TecnoLógicas. 2023;26(57):e2731.
11. Tang X, Wang B, Rong Y. Artificial intelligence will reduce the need for clinical medical physicists. J Appl Clin Med Phys. 2018;19(1):6–9.
12. Abdullah A, Bangcola A. Investigating the perspectives of millennial and gen Z nurses on quiet quitting in Marawi City, Lanao del Sur. Philippines Malays J Nurs. 2024;16(01):135–48.
13. Labrague LJ, Al Sabei S, Al Rawajfah O, Burney I, AbuAlRub R. Gen Z nurses: examining the direct and indirect effects of job burnout on work satisfaction and the mediating role of the nurse work environment. Worldviews Evid-Based Nurs. 2025;22(3):e70038.

Cutting Edge Exemplars and Promising Practices

8

Rachel Cox Simms , Karen Hunt , and Rebecca Hill

8.1 Introduction

As artificial intelligence rapidly transforms healthcare delivery, nursing professionals face both unprecedented opportunities and critical challenges. This chapter examines the responsible integration of AI across nursing education and clinical practice through six evidence-based case studies. Each exemplar demonstrates practical AI applications while addressing essential safety, equity, and ethical considerations. By exploring both successes and limitations, this chapter provides guidance for implementing AI tools that enhance nursing practice without compromising the profession's core values of patient-centered care, clinical judgment, and human connection. The case studies that follow are fictional composites. Although each scenario is informed by real-world lessons and professional experience, no single patient, institution, or published project is portrayed. The vignettes are offered solely to illustrate possibilities, provoke discussion, and inspire innovation—not to report empirical results.

R. C. Simms (✉) · K. Hunt
MGH Institute of Health Professions, Boston, MA, USA
e-mail: rlcox@mghihp.edu; klhunt@mghihp.edu

R. Hill
University of North Carolina at Chapel Hill, Chapel Hill, NC, USA
e-mail: rebecca.hill@unc.edu

D. W. La Rosa et al. (eds.), *Nursing Education in the AI Era*,
https://doi.org/10.1007/978-3-032-12402-9_8

8.1.1 Case Study Exemplar 1: AI-Generated NCLEX-Style Question Bank

8.1.1.1 Background and Context

Dr. Sarah Johnson (she/her), an assistant professor in the prelicensure nursing program at Riverbend University, has long balanced high enrollment (120 students per cohort) with limited faculty bandwidth. Historically, she devoted 10–15 hours each semester to craft and refine NCLEX-style questions, time that increasingly competed with her teaching and student-mentoring responsibilities.

This semester, she discovered that several students had obtained old exams from prior years, compromising the integrity of her existing test bank. At the same time, the NCLEX Test Plan was updated and a new third edition of the med-surg textbook was released, making it critical to generate fresh items that reflect current guidelines and content.

In preparing to pilot generative AI, Dr. Johnson reviewed a recent study, which demonstrated that with targeted prompts and rigorous faculty review, ChatGPT can produce NCLEX items matching human-authored questions in clarity, clinical accuracy, and cognitive complexity [1]. Bolstered by those findings, Dr. Johnson felt confident moving forward with an AI-assisted workflow, provided that human oversight remained central.

8.1.1.2 Implementation

Dr. Johnson mapped her question bank to the NCLEX Test Plan, focusing on areas where students performed poorly: acid-base balance, fluid/electrolyte management, and patient safety. She aimed to create application-level multiple-choice questions with one correct answer and three plausible distractors.

She developed standardized prompt templates incorporating clinical vignettes, patient demographics, learning objectives, and formatting rules. For example: "Create an NCLEX-style question on interpreting ABG results for a patient with Kussmaul respirations. Include one correct answer identifying the primary acid-base disturbance and three distractors reflecting common misinterpretations."

Running 20-prompt batches through ChatGPT yielded 80 draft items per session. After discarding 10% for inaccuracies or hallucinated content, Dr. Johnson and her co-teacher refined the remaining questions in one-hour validation sessions (checking clinical accuracy, adjusting distractors, and ensuring cultural inclusivity), consistently producing 60 high-quality questions.

8.1.1.3 Hypothetical Outcomes and Evaluation

For the purposes of this fictitious case study, results showed dramatic efficiency gains: drafting time dropped from 12 to 2 hours per 60-item set. Including 4 hours for editing/validation, Dr. Johnson saved 6 hours per semester. Student quiz averages improved from 78% to 84%, and 92% of 110 surveyed students found the AI-generated questions "clear, realistic, and clinically relevant." Most importantly, reduced "exam-prep burnout" allowed Dr. Johnson to focus more on individual student coaching.

8.1.1.4 Challenges and Barriers

The implementation faced several challenges. Initial AI outputs occasionally included "hallucinated" information about outdated protocols, requiring careful screening. The technology demanded significant upfront investment in prompt engineering and template refinement. Faculty time for validation remained essential, as the AI could not replace human expertise in ensuring clinical accuracy and educational appropriateness. Additionally, ensuring diverse representation in patient scenarios required conscious effort and regular auditing.

8.1.1.5 Lessons Learned

The use of AI to generate an NCLEX test bank can decrease the total amount of time required to create NCLEX items and help maintain exam integrity, provided that oversight by a nurse educator is maintained. AI can help ensure alignment with best practice in NCLEX items, evidence-based practice, and textbook materials. However, there is a risk of bias with the use of AI-generated NCLEX-type questions; linguistic inclusivity and incorporating representation across diverse patient populations are paramount [2]. Faculty expertise is required to validate the accuracy, level of difficulty in association with the course level, and fairness of AI-generated items [2].

8.1.2 Case Study Exemplar 2: AI-Enhanced Case Study Assignment in Nursing Education

8.1.2.1 Background and Context

Dr. Emily Carter (she/her), an associate professor in the prelicensure nursing program at Westlake College of Health Sciences, faced a familiar challenge: finding new ways to teach critical thinking, clinical judgment, and information literacy in an era where students increasingly relied on generative AI.

Recent incidents highlighted concerns: several students submitted discussion posts heavily AI-generated without proper evaluation or critical engagement. Inspired by the strategies outlined in a recent paper, Dr. Carter decided to turn AI into an educational scaffold rather than a shortcut, helping students develop essential skills to critically appraise and refine AI-generated material [3].

8.1.2.2 Implementation

Dr. Carter created a multi-phase assignment where students used ChatGPT to generate a clinical case study for a patient with multiple comorbidities (diabetes, heart failure, kidney disease), then critically evaluated the output for accuracy, realism, bias, and evidence-based alignment.

Students revised and annotated the AI-generated cases, noting inaccuracies and missing information, then reflected on AI's benefits and limitations. Dr. Carter provided structured prompts, such as "Generate a detailed case study for a 68-year-old male with heart failure and diabetes. Include realistic clinical data and three nursing decision points."

The assignment progressed through four phases: AI generation, critical appraisal against clinical guidelines, case refinement with citations, and reflective analysis. Students used a comprehensive checklist to assess clinical accuracy, demographic inclusivity, and ethical considerations.

A case critique workshop allowed students to share common AI issues (hallucinated medications, missing psychosocial context, unrealistic vital signs) reinforcing critical appraisal skills and building a community of responsible AI practice.

8.1.2.3 Hypothetical Outcomes and Evaluation

For the purposes of this fictitious case study, students showed remarkable skill development after the assignment, particularly in identifying clinical inaccuracies in AI content. Many reported feeling "more confident" evaluating AI-generated information, with subsequent work demonstrating enhanced critical thinking. Students now automatically questioned sources and verified clinical data against evidence-based guidelines.

Engagement increased notably, with students feeling empowered to question rather than accepting AI outputs without careful consideration. Many recognized these skills as crucial for future practice. As one student noted, "I used to think AI had all the answers. Now I see it as a tool that needs my nursing knowledge to be useful."

Dr. Carter observed lasting benefits: students' case studies and care plans showed increased depth throughout the course, suggesting AI critique skills transferred to other work. This structured AI integration addressed academic integrity concerns without requiring technology bans.

8.1.2.4 Challenges and Barriers

Implementation wasn't without obstacles. The varying levels of AI literacy among students created some initial disparities. Some students struggled to generate useful outputs while others needed guidance in maintaining appropriate skepticism. Technical challenges arose when the AI platform experienced intermittent outages during assignment periods, requiring contingency planning.

Students initially showed resistance to the additional work of critiquing AI output, with some questioning why they couldn't simply use AI-generated content directly. This required careful explanation of the assignment's learning objectives and its relevance to their future practice. Time management proved challenging for some students who underestimated the effort required for thorough critique and revision of AI-generated cases.

8.1.2.5 Lessons Learned

Teaching students to critique AI output is an essential component to the development of critical thinking, clinical judgment, and digital literacy. This is a requisite for the continued use of AI in nursing practice as students transition into the nursing workforce. AI can be a creative use of a scaffolded approach to learning; it should never be used as a shortcut or definitive answer to nursing practice. The differing levels of AI-literacy in students may highlight opportunity gaps. Similar to how we evaluate Social Determinants of Health (SDOH) in patient care, the Social Determinants of Learning (SDOL) must be considered for students [4]. Educators must realize that accessibility to AI tools is not always equitable; accessibility to devices, internet connectivity, and the presence of language barriers should be considered prior to implementation in the educational setting. The increased presence of AI in higher education is unavoidable. Academic integrity can be maintained through the guided use of AI, and students should be encouraged to be transparent in their use of AI for assistance with coursework.

8.1.3 Case Study Exemplar 3: AI-Enhanced Simulation Scenario Design and Debriefing

8.1.3.1 Background and Context

Dr. Jeff Martinez (he/him), Director of Simulation Education in the prelicensure nursing program at Meadowbrook University, oversees six high-fidelity simulation sessions each semester. Crafting each scenario (patient profiles, vital-sign trajectories, moulage notes, and debriefing guides) used to consume 15–20 faculty hours. Meanwhile, students reported inconsistent scenario complexity and limited opportunities to reflect on both clinical decision-making and emerging digital tools in healthcare.

To streamline development and introduce students to critical evaluation of AI-generated content, Dr. Martinez piloted a workflow using ChatGPT to draft initial scenario scripts, branching decision points, and debrief questions, while building in student-led critique of those AI outputs as part of their simulation literacy curriculum [5].

8.1.3.2 Implementation

Dr. Martinez piloted AI-assisted simulation design focusing on high-stakes scenarios: COPD exacerbation, postoperative hemorrhage, and sepsis recognition. He developed detailed prompts for comprehensive simulation scripts, such as "Generate a high-fidelity simulation for a 68-year-old patient with COPD with increased work of breathing. Include: 5-step vital sign progression, standardized-patient dialogue, two branching decision points, required props, and five debriefing questions."

Before engaging students in the process, they completed mandatory HIPAA training, learning to create fully de-identified scenarios and understanding that inputting real patient data would constitute serious violations. Final scenarios were loaded into simulation software with time-stamped cues. During sessions, faculty triggered mannequin changes following AI-generated vital-sign progressions, creating dynamic scenarios that challenged clinical reasoning.

Implementation combined faculty review with student co-creation. Dr. Martinez corrected AI errors like inappropriate SpO_2 thresholds, while Year-3 nursing students in workshops generated alternative scenarios, compared versions, identified AI "hallucinations" and submitted improved prompts and error logs for credit.

8.1.3.3 Hypothetical Outcomes and Evaluation

For the purposes of this fictitious case study, the pilot program delivered exceptional efficiency gains, cutting scenario development time from 18 hours to just 5 hours per scenario, including student workshops. This improvement enabled more frequent scenario refreshes and development of additional scenarios for emerging clinical challenges.

The majority of faculty rated the AI-drafted scripts as "usable with minor edits" compared to the initial manual drafts. Most edits focused on clinical timing (adjusting response intervals to match real-world scenarios), cultural appropriateness (ensuring diverse patient representations), and standardized patient coaching notes. AI excelled at consistent formatting, logical vital sign progressions, and comprehensive equipment lists, though human expertise remained crucial for clinical nuance and emotional authenticity. Faculty reported spending roughly 60% less time on revisions compared to refining manually-drafted scenarios.

Student outcomes exceeded expectations: most reported that critiquing AI outputs deepened their understanding of simulation design and clinical judgment. Reflective journals showed improved ability to spot subtle flaws like unrealistic timing or missing cultural considerations. Students gained sophisticated insights into simulation construction, leading to more thoughtful future participation.

8.1.3.4 Challenges and Barriers

Technical challenges emerged throughout implementation. The AI occasionally generated clinically impossible scenarios, such as normal arterial blood gases despite severe respiratory distress. Prompt engineering required significant refinement to achieve consistent quality outputs. The AI struggled with emotional nuance, often producing standardized-patient dialogue that sounded robotic or failed to capture the authentic distress of acutely ill patients.

Faculty resistance initially posed obstacles, with some simulation specialists concerned that AI-generated scenarios lacked the intuitive understanding that experienced educators bring to scenario design. Student workload increased during the pilot phase as they participated in scenario critique workshops in addition to regular simulation sessions. Integration with existing simulation management software required technical support and workflow adjustments.

8.1.3.5 Lessons Learned

In this scenario, Dr. Martinez was able to accelerate simulation design using AI. In using this tool, Dr. Martinez may have improved his digital tool utilization and enhanced his simulation literacy with the different iterations created. However, it is important to remember that it is common for AI to limit the incorporation of cultural sensitivity or diverse patient populations in simulation scenarios. The ethical and inclusive use of AI can be discussed with students, with prompts that encourage them to identify and address such gaps. Faculty oversight and expertise are imperative to ensure alignment with student learning outcomes, appropriate leveling of the content and performance expectations based on the course where it falls in the curriculum, and professional nursing standards.

8.1.4   Case Study Exemplar 4: AI Scribe for Documentation

8.1.4.1 Background and Context

Tyler De Luca (they/them) is a family nurse practitioner working in a busy primary care clinic, where they are expected to see 14–18 patients per day while staying on a tight schedule. Many of the patients served at this clinic present with complex medical and social needs. Emotional responses during visits are common, especially as treatment plans are initiated or changed, requiring Tyler to respond with empathy and compassion. This often limits their ability to complete documentation in real time.

In addition to patient care, Tyler frequently works late to complete prior authorizations and spends evenings preparing for the next day's appointments. These extended hours, filled with documentation and administrative tasks, are contributing to feelings of burnout. Tyler remains committed to providing high-quality, patient-centered care but wishes they could spend more time connecting with patients and less time behind a computer.

8.1.4.2 Implementation

After speaking with colleagues who shared similar documentation challenges, Tyler approached the clinic's medical director to propose a potential solution: an AI-powered ambient scribe tool that captures provider-patient interactions through voice recognition [6]. The medical director approved a six-week pilot using secure, HIPAA-compliant software integrated into the electronic health record (EHR) with three providers, including Tyler. The AI system transcribed real-time conversations and narrated clinical observations directly into the EHR. Providers reviewed and edited the notes before finalizing them. Feedback was collected through focus groups and documentation audits to evaluate usability and effectiveness.

8.1.4.3 Hypothetical Outcomes and Evaluation

For the purposes of this fictitious case study, at the end of the six-week pilot, all three participating providers reported a noticeable reduction in documentation time. Tyler estimated saving an average of 45–60 minutes per day, allowing for more focused patient interactions and fewer after-hours tasks.

Documentation metrics reflected these improvements, with a marked increase in the percentage of notes closed on the same day and a decrease in average after-work time spent on charting. Focus group feedback highlighted improved workflow efficiency and reduced documentation-related stress. Providers found the tool especially helpful in capturing detailed subjective information during emotionally complex encounters. However, they emphasized the importance of carefully reviewing AI-generated documentation, as occasional misinterpretations did occur.

Documentation audits confirmed that notes remained complete and met clinical quality standards. While the tool did not offer a fully keyboard-free experience, it was widely perceived as a valuable support that preserved provider autonomy and alleviated some administrative burden. Based on these results, the medical director began exploring expansion of the tool to additional providers and integrating AI support into onboarding and training processes.

8.1.4.4 Challenges and Barriers

Despite overall success, implementation faced several obstacles. Technical challenges included occasional speech recognition errors, particularly with medical terminology or accented speech. The AI sometimes struggled with complex patient presentations involving multiple complaints or nonlinear narratives. Initial setup required significant time investment for voice training and customization to individual provider styles.

Provider adaptation varied, with some requiring multiple sessions to develop fluency with the voice-narration workflow. Concerns arose about the AI's ability to accurately capture nonverbal communication and emotional nuance. Some providers worried about becoming overly dependent on the technology, potentially affecting their documentation skills during system outages or when caring for patients who declined recording.

Patient-related challenges included occasional discomfort with recording despite consent procedures. Some patients became self-conscious knowing their words were being transcribed, potentially affecting the authenticity of their communication. The team also encountered situations where family members present during visits had different comfort levels with recording than the patients themselves.

8.1.4.5 Lessons Learned

In this case, we learned that AI can reduce provider burnout and improve patient care [6]. Tyler's use of AI reduced after-hours charting and more time during the clinical shift was available for direct patient care and interaction. There were also fewer errors in documentation. With AI-generated documentation, there are important challenges and considerations to take into account. AI can create bias in speech recognition that can lead to inaccurate or incomplete documentation. AI scribes can be costly and as such, will not be accessible in limited-resource settings. Patients may not be comfortable with voice recording; consent should be obtained prior to use.

In the area of inclusive practice, AI may default to heteronormative assumptions. Misgendering can harm the nurse-patient relationship and damage trust [7]. Emotions, facial expressions, and cultural differences can be missed when using AI. Providers must continue to review transcripts of documentation to ensure accuracy and the incorporation of these nuances. These AI errors can also lead to clinical harm, HIPAA-related breaches, and situations around patient autonomy [8]. Real-time editing and thorough review, HIPAA-compliant software, and informed consent prior to use are essential considerations for the ethical use of AI for documentation in the health record.

Based on these challenges, responsible use of AI in healthcare and healthcare education should include:

1. Piloting use with diverse speech patterns and dialects.
2. Building consent into the clinical workflow.

3. Training AI to recognize gender-inclusive language.
4. Reflecting on the ethical considerations of AI.
5. Considering how the patient felt about the use of this tool for documentation.

8.1.5 Case Study Exemplar 5: Early Sepsis Detection

8.1.5.1 Background and Context

On a busy Friday afternoon, Diane Lee, a 72-year-old woman (she/her), arrived at the emergency department at 15:30 with her partner. Her chief complaint was weakness and a fall at home without head strike or loss of consciousness. The triage nurse noted confusion, elevated heart rate, and slight fever, initially attributing symptoms to anxiety and possible dehydration. Head CT ruled out trauma from the fall.

Past medical history included type 2 diabetes and hypertension. Initial assessment revealed: temperature 38.2 °C, heart rate 112 bpm, respiratory rate 22/min, blood pressure 102/68 mmHg, SpO2 94% on room air, and pain 3/10 in lower abdomen. The patient was alert and oriented to person and place but confused about time. Physical exam showed warm, flushed skin, fine crackles in bilateral lung bases, sinus tachycardia, and tenderness to lower abdominal palpation.

Jamie Wilcox, RN, assumed care of Diane in the emergency department, placing her on cardiac monitoring, obtaining IV access, and initiating laboratory studies including complete blood count, basic metabolic panel, lactate, and blood cultures. A chest X-ray was ordered and IV fluids started at 100 mL/hr. The emergency department had recently implemented an AI-based clinical decision support system designed to identify patients at risk for sepsis by continuously analyzing vital signs, laboratory values, and clinical data patterns [9].

8.1.5.2 Implementation

Three hours into Diane's ED stay, her condition subtly deteriorated. Vital signs showed temperature rising to 38.5 °C, heart rate 118 bpm, respiratory rate 24/min, blood pressure dropping to 98/64 mmHg, and SpO2 92% on room air. Laboratory results revealed elevated white blood cell count of 16,200, lactate of 2.6 mmol/L, creatinine of 1.6 mg/dL, and glucose of 186 mg/dL.

As Jamie prepared to review the new data, an alert appeared on the EHR screen: "CLINICAL DECISION SUPPORT ALERT: Patient parameters indicate potential infection with systemic involvement. Consider sepsis protocol evaluation." The AI-based risk analysis system had integrated multiple data points (vital sign trends, laboratory values, and patient demographics) to identify a pattern consistent with developing sepsis.

Jamie clicked on the alert for additional information and found specific risk factors highlighted: upward trending temperature and heart rate, elevated lactate, new acute kidney injury, and the patient's age placing her at higher risk. The system recommended immediate actions including repeat lactate within one hour, blood cultures before antibiotics, broad-spectrum antibiotic administration within three hours, and aggressive fluid resuscitation.

Returning immediately to Diane's bedside, Jamie noted her mental status had deteriorated further and extremities were now cool despite fever. Jamie notified the provider urgently, and new orders were implemented: blood cultures drawn, broad-spectrum antibiotics initiated, IV fluid rate increased, urine obtained via catheterization for culture, chest X-ray changed to STAT, and repeat lactate ordered.

8.1.5.3 Hypothetical Outcomes and Evaluation

For the purposes of this fictitious case study, the prompt recognition and early intervention proved crucial. By hour six, Diane's lactate had decreased to 1.4 mmol/L, blood pressure stabilized at 110/72 mmHg, and mental status began improving. Urine cultures later confirmed E. coli as the causative organism, allowing antibiotics to be narrowed based on sensitivities. The early sepsis bundle implementation (a standardized set of time-sensitive treatments including antibiotics, blood cultures, and IV fluids) likely prevented progression to septic shock and ICU transfer.

The ED's metrics showed improvement after AI implementation: door-to-antibiotic time for sepsis patients decreased from 185 to 97 minutes on average, and sepsis-related mortality dropped by 18% over six months. Nursing staff reported increased confidence in identifying subtle signs of clinical deterioration. However, alarm fatigue (where clinicians become desensitized to frequent system notifications) emerged as a concern, with the system generating false positives in approximately 15% of cases.

8.1.5.4 Lessons Learned

Diane's case illustrates how AI can enhance timely care and improve patient outcomes. Using the AI-based risk analysis in the clinical workflow prompted Jamie to reassess, follow protocols, and provide earlier intervention, thus leading to stabilizing the patient. Despite this excellent utilization of AI, clinical judgment remains an essential component of nursing care. Jamie's prompt attention to the change in Diane's condition and prompt reassessment was critical. The combination between clinical expertise and AI support produces the most optimal outcome. Seamless integration within the EHR makes AI tools usable, actionable, and can increase the uptake of use by clinicians across healthcare disciplines.

It is important to acknowledge the risk of bias in AI training data. AI models may mis- or under-represent marginalized populations or those with complex health situations or comorbidities [10]. In this exemplar, patients like Diane (elderly, female, co-morbid diabetes) could be overlooked or underemphasized. AI tends to exclude SDOH data [10]. Things such as access to healthcare, food insecurity, and insurance status may not be considered; these critical factors in the holistic understanding of health status and their associations with access to care may not be captured. AI lacks the ability to assess nonverbal signs of illness and could fail to incorporate cultural differences. It is important to generate case studies that represent diversity of patients and populations to promote inclusive teaching and emphasize equity-informed clinical reasoning and nursing practice. Similarly, the ethical and appropriate use of AI must not be understated. It is imperative that clinical training continue at the highest quality so that nurses can interpret and validate AI prompts and alerts with confidence. Patients should be informed when AI is being used in the determination of clinical care decision-making. Lastly, responsibility will always remain with the clinical care team. As such, when AI generates an incorrect answer or delivers the wrong treatment recommendation, the healthcare team will need to identify those errors and act using their vast knowledge and clinical reasoning.

Recommendations for building AI-based case studies in a responsible way include:

1. Check for inclusion of equity flags.
   (a) What SDOH may alter the course of this situation?
   (b) Who may not be considered with this AI tool?
2. Build narratives that represent diverse patients.
   (a) Feature patients that vary in age, race, gender, disability status.
3. Promote ethical reflection.
   (a) Is AI negatively affecting patient autonomy?
4. Develop sound rationale for the use or disregard for the AI recommendations.
   (a) Do the recommendations align with best practice?

8.1.6 Case Study Exemplar 6: Machine Learning for Fall Prevention

8.1.6.1 Background and Context

Randall Douglass, a 77-year-old man (he/him), was admitted to a medical/surgical unit for heart failure exacerbation. He presented with dyspnea, lower extremity edema, four-pillow orthopnea, and recent weight gain. His medical history included hypertension, heart failure, hypercholesterolemia, and stage 2 chronic kidney disease. Treatment included IV diuretics, oxygen therapy, sodium restriction, and strict fluid monitoring.

Living alone with support from nearby family, Mr. Douglass had become increasingly forgetful over the past year. His children reported better cognitive function in mornings but concerning confusion during evenings. Two unwitnessed falls in six months, though without major injury, hadn't convinced him to use assistive devices. He valued independence and privacy deeply, expressing to the social worker his difficulty accepting help and desire to be "left in peace."

Nursing assessment revealed orthostatic vital sign changes, occasional premature ventricular contractions (PVCs) on telemetry, and significant activity intolerance. His Morse Fall Scale score of 101 indicated high fall risk. Despite standard precautions (bed alarms, lowered bed position, visible signage, and reminders to call for assistance) Mr. Douglass often overestimated his abilities and attempted unassisted transfers.

8.1.6.2 Implementation

As the day nurse prepared for shift change, staffing shortages for the evening shift raised concerns about Mr. Douglass's safety. The unit was participating in a pilot program using AI-powered camera monitoring systems that detected movement patterns indicating fall risk [11, 12]. These privacy-preserving sensors captured only depth and motion data without identifiable images.

After discussing Mr. Douglass's independence needs and safety requirements, the resource nurse and bedside nurse agreed to activate the AI monitoring system for his room beginning that evening. The technology provided graduated responses to unsafe movements: first, a gentle voice reminder through the room speaker, then staff alerts if risky behavior continued.

During implementation, the nursing team faced the delicate balance of respecting Mr. Douglass's autonomy while ensuring safety. They positioned the technology as a support system rather than surveillance, though notably failed to obtain explicit consent or inform his family, a decision that would later prove problematic.

8.1.6.3 Hypothetical Outcomes and Evaluation

For the purposes of this fictitious case study, throughout the evening and night shifts, the AI system prevented three potential falls by detecting high-risk movement patterns before balance was lost. The technology identified subtle pre-fall behaviors: weight shifting toward bed edges, unstable standing attempts, and gait patterns associated with imminent falls. Staff responded to alerts within 90 seconds on average, arriving before falls occurred.

The next morning, Mr. Douglass hadn't experienced any falls, and his daughter arrived for her visit. Upon noticing the ceiling-mounted sensors, she immediately expressed concern to the nurse director: "Why wasn't our family informed about this monitoring system?" Despite explanations about privacy safeguards and successful fall prevention, the family remained troubled by the lack of explicit consent.

Unit-wide metrics showed 40% reduction in fall rates during the pilot period. However, implementation inconsistencies emerged, with some rooms having better sensor positioning than others. Staff response times varied significantly based on workload and competing priorities.

8.1.6.4 Challenges and Barriers

The fall prevention system faced interconnected barriers spanning patient acceptance, technical limitations, and staffing realities. Patient acceptance proved challenging, as several patients like Mr. Douglass viewed monitoring as threatening their independence and dignity, with some requesting sensor deactivation despite fall risk. Technical limitations compounded these concerns. The system couldn't distinguish between intentional movement (reaching for water) and unsafe attempts (trying to stand alone), leading to frequent false alarms that further frustrated patients.

Infrastructure constraints created additional complications. Blind spots in bathrooms for privacy protection ironically excluded areas where many falls occur, while the AI struggled with low lighting conditions common during night shifts. Integration with existing call bell systems proved complex, requiring workarounds that confused staff and undermined system efficiency.

These technical issues intersected with staffing challenges in problematic ways. Nurses reported alarm fatigue from frequent alerts, while some worried the technology might justify further staffing reductions. Training requirements added to workload during an already challenging staffing situation, creating a paradoxical effect where the fall prevention system initially worsened staffing stress rather than alleviating it.

8.1.6.5 Lessons Learned

The implementation of fall prevention technology using AI requires consideration of both patient consent and autonomy. The introduction of technologies such as these should include communication, education, and collaboration. While the use of AI to predict and prevent falls can enhance patient safety, it is not a replacement for clinical care and already established practices such as patient rounding, shift reports, and the use of other patient-centered practices (e.g., bed alarms, intentional bed assignment near the nurses' station).

Barriers to using this type of technology include issues around patient privacy and resistance to acceptance by the patient. In the case of Mr. Douglass, he was resistant to these interventions as they were perceived as a threat to his privacy. If the unit is understaffed, there may be a reliance on AI technology, and the fall prevention practices may be underutilized. As with any other technology, training and acceptance from the staff is a requisite to use. Just as the incorporation of the EHR has demonstrated, these technologies may also reduce the human connection between nurse and patient. Care should be taken to maintain interaction and direct care.

Despite these potential barriers, the AI monitoring system effectively prevented three falls. The voice reminders and real-time AI monitoring allowed for faster and more precise nursing interventions. During a time of staffing limitations, this technology contributed to patient safety and fall prevention.

The use of AI for fall prevention can be a useful tool, provided certain recommendations are in place. First, consent for use should be explicit and incorporated into the admission protocol for patients classified as high risk of falling. The purpose of the technology should be discussed with both the patient and their family. Patient preferences for use, along with the maintenance of patient dignity and autonomy must be ensured. The technology must be HIPAA compliant and used as a supplement, not replacement, to patient care. Collaboration with information technology, ethics committees, and leadership should be considered, along with an established process to evaluate quality improvement initiatives that use AI in patient care.

8.1.7 Ethics, Safety, and Equity Considerations

As artificial intelligence becomes increasingly integrated into nursing education and clinical practice, it brings substantial benefits such as enhanced efficiency, improved patient safety, and enriched learning experiences. However, these advancements are accompanied by critical considerations related to safety, equity, and ethics. Effective integration of AI demands careful attention to risks such as misinformation, biases, and inequitable access to technology, as well as the ethical implications of autonomy, consent, and privacy. The following table (Table 8.1) succinctly outlines these key considerations across various AI implementation exemplars, highlighting essential factors for responsible and inclusive use.

Table 8.1 Key ethics, safety, and equity considerations for responsible and inclusive AI use

Exemplar	Safety considerations	Equity considerations	Ethical considerations
NCLEX question bank	Ensuring accurate, clinically appropriate items through faculty validation. Avoiding misinformation from AI hallucinations.	AI defaults can overlook diversity unless specifically prompted, requiring deliberate inclusivity checks. Linguistic accessibility important for diverse student populations.	Human oversight necessary to maintain educational integrity. Risks of bias and misrepresentation require active mitigation.
Case study assignment	Ensuring clinical accuracy by critical student and faculty review of AI-generated content. Risk of students uncritically accepting AI output.	Accessibility disparities due to unequal technology access among students. AI may perpetuate biases in patient scenarios without deliberate checks.	Importance of transparency in student AI use for academic integrity. Training students to ethically critique and improve AI-generated content.
Simulation scenario	Risk of clinically unrealistic scenarios generated by AI, potentially compromising training effectiveness. Need for careful review to maintain scenario authenticity and patient safety.	Training datasets may lack diversity, resulting in scenarios less relevant to underrepresented groups. Accessibility issues for students without equal AI access.	HIPAA compliance critical to protect patient information. Student training on ethical implications of AI in patient data handling.
AI scribe documentation	Risks of transcription errors leading to clinical mistakes. Providers must carefully review notes to ensure safety.	Speech recognition inaccuracies disproportionately affect accented speech, leading to inequitable documentation quality. Financial accessibility issues in resource-limited settings.	Informed patient consent essential for AI recording. Privacy concerns related to handling sensitive patient data and voice recordings. Ethical use of patient narratives and authenticity of clinical records.

(continued)

Table 8.1 (continued)

Exemplar	Safety considerations	Equity considerations	Ethical considerations
Early sepsis detection	Enhances early identification of clinical deterioration and timely intervention. Risks include alert fatigue and false positives leading to unnecessary interventions.	AI trained on less diverse data may miss atypical presentations common in underrepresented populations. Language barriers may reduce effective use.	Clinical judgment must remain primary. Importance of patient informed consent when AI supports clinical decisions. Ethical implications of relying solely on AI for critical decision-making.
Machine learning for fall prevention	AI enhances patient safety by predicting and preventing falls. Potential risks include reliance on technology and alarm fatigue.	Monitoring effectiveness varies across different patient demographics and body types. Inequitable distribution of AI resources due to cost constraints.	Explicit patient and family consent crucial. Privacy concerns regarding continual monitoring. Balancing safety benefits with patient autonomy and dignity.

8.2 Conclusions

The case studies above demonstrate AI's transformative potential in nursing education and practice, from enhancing patient safety through early sepsis detection to improving educational efficiency through automated content generation. AI has shown measurable benefits: reducing documentation time, preventing falls, accelerating curriculum development, and supporting clinical decision-making.

However, responsible implementation requires addressing critical challenges:

- Bias and equity: AI systems trained on limited datasets may perpetuate healthcare disparities.
- Over-reliance risks: Technology cannot replace clinical judgment or holistic nursing care.
- Privacy and consent: Patient autonomy must be protected through transparent communication.
- Quality assurance: Human oversight remains essential to validate AI outputs.

Success depends on viewing AI as a tool to augment, not replace, nursing expertise. By maintaining focus on patient-centered care, ensuring inclusive design, and preserving the human elements of nursing practice, we can harness AI's benefits while upholding our profession's core values.

AI Disclosure
ChatGPT-4.0 (OpenAI) was used during the development of this manuscript to assist with brainstorming, editing, and revising text. All content was reviewed and finalized by the authors to ensure accuracy and integrity.

References

1. Cox RL, Hunt KL, Hill RR. Comparative analysis of NCLEX-RN questions: a duel between CHATGPT and human expertise. J Nurs Educ. 2023;62(12):679–87. https://doi.org/10.3928/01484834-20231006-07.
2. García-Rudolph A, Sanchez-Pinsach D, Fernandez-Mira C, Cunyat S, Opisso E, Hernandez-Pena E. Accuracy analysis of AI chatbots GPT-3.5 and GEMINI on English NCLEX-style and Spanish EU general nursing multiple choice questions: challenges and performance insights Teach Learn Nurs [Internet]. 2025 Jul 1 [cited 2025 Jun 12];20(3):e730–e735. Available from: https://research-ebsco-com.treadwell.idm.oclc.org/linkprocessor/plink?id=f7c83055-328c-3889-830d-aff40f9811703
3. Simms RC. Work with CHATGPT, not against: 3 teaching strategies that harness the power of artificial intelligence. Nurse Educ. 2024;49(3):158–61. https://doi.org/10.1097/nne.0000000000001634.
4. Sanderson CD, Hollinger-Smith LM, Cox K. Developing a social determinants of Learning™ Framework: a case study. Nursing Education Perspectives (Wolters Kluwer Health) [Internet]. 2021 Jul 1 [cited 2025 Jun 12];42(4):205–211. Available from: https://research-ebsco-com.treadwell.idm.oclc.org/linkprocessor/plink?id=e9e6683c-e5bf-335c-9618-dbc3b1ab76d9
5. Chan MM, Wan AW, Cheung DS, Choi EP, Chan EA, Yorke J, et al. Integration of artificial intelligence in nursing simulation education. Nurse Educ. 2025; https://doi.org/10.1097/nne.0000000000001851.
6. Duggan MJ, Gervase J, Schoenbaum A, Hanson W, Howell JT, Sheinberg M, et al. Clinician experiences with ambient scribe technology to assist with documentation burden and efficiency. JAMA Netw Open. 2025;8(2) https://doi.org/10.1001/jamanetworkopen.2024.60637.
7. Gomez AM, Hooker N, Olip-Booth R, Woerner P, Ratliff GA. "It's being compassionate, not making assumptions": transmasculine and nonbinary young adults' experiences of "women's" health care settings. Womens Health Issues [Internet]. 2021 Jul 1 [cited 2025 Jun 12];31(4):324–331. Available from: https://research-ebsco-com.treadwell.idm.oclc.org/linkprocessor/plink?id=07a03839-ab8c-3619-ac0d-de7e30d49775
8. Hoelscher SH. The good, the bad, and the binary: ethical impact of AI on nursing practice. Nursing [Internet]. 2025 Apr 1 [cited 2025 Jun 12];55(4):26–32. https://doi.org/10.1097/NSG.0000000000000160.
9. Boussina A, Shashikumar SP, Malhotra A, Owens RL, El-Kareh R, Longhurst CA, et al. Impact of a deep learning sepsis prediction model on quality of care and survival. NPJ Digital Med. 2024;7(1) https://doi.org/10.1038/s41746-023-00986-6.
10. Cross JL, Choma MA, Onofrey JA. Bias in medical AI: implications for clinical decision-making. PLoS Digit Health [Internet]. 2024 Nov 7 [cited 2025 Jun 12];3(11):1–19. Available from: https://research-ebsco-com.treadwell.idm.oclc.org/linkprocessor/plink?id=a56f9f00-1031-3df9-9e45-58d30b9b66d7
11. O'Connor S, Gasteiger N, Stanmore E, Wong DC, Lee JJ. Artificial intelligence for falls management in older adult care: a scoping review of nurses' role. J Nurs Manag. 2022;30(8):3787–801. https://doi.org/10.1111/jonm.13853.
12. Riviera DF, Morelli JD, Barrett-Fajardo N, Mattia A, Mcdonough KA. Transforming the paradigm of care to reduce falls on a medical-surgical unit using artificial intelligence. [Internet]. [cited 2025 May 12]. Available from: https://www.thefreelibrary.com/Transforming the Paradigm of Care to Reduce Falls on a...-a0765867278

Nursing Education in the AI Era: A Summary

Antonia M. Villarruel

The AI revolution is transforming all aspects of healthcare and is similarly changing nursing education and practice. While technology is evolving at a rapid pace, the cohesive and forward-thinking guidance in the chapters of *Nursing Education in the AI Era: Practical Guidance for Educators to Provide Equitable Care* offers a solid foundation for teaching that transcends inevitable changes in technology and practice. This foundation includes embracing AI and technology, fostering digital literacy, strengthening core nursing skills, and cultivating innovation and leadership in technology use.

Embracing AI and Technology The challenge ahead is not "if" we will use AI, but "how" we will use it to enhance learning and prepare competent and safe nurses. Like any innovation, AI holds both promise and peril. In clinical settings AI holds much promise, for example, in reducing administrative burdens such as documentation of patient-clinician encounters, synthesizing multiple sources of data, such as patient monitoring, and identifying and proposing treatment options with the use of decision support systems. However, concerns include overreliance on AI systems, diminishing use of clinical reasoning and judgement, algorithmic bias that perpetuates disparities in treatment, and ethical issues, such as data privacy. In education, AI enables opportunities for personalized and equitable learning experiences but also raises concerns about academic integrity and diminished critical thinking.

Fostering Digital Literacy Digital literacy is essential for educators, clinicians, and students to effectively use and design AI. AI literacy involves knowledge and critical analysis of the application of AI outputs and tools, including clinical decision support systems and remote patient monitoring to improve patient outcomes, workflow optimization to increase efficiency and reduce costs, and patient safety, all of which needs to occur within an ethical framework (Chapter 4, 2025). Understanding the benefits and limitations of AI-generated data and the application

A. M. Villarruel
Office of the Dean, University of Pennsylvania School of Nursing, Philadelphia, PA, USA
e-mail: nursingdean@nursing.upenn.edu; amvillar@nursing.upenn.edu

D. W. La Rosa et al. (eds.), *Nursing Education in the AI Era*,
https://doi.org/10.1007/978-3-032-12402-9

157

of AI-assisted clinical decision-making tools are important skills to be developed (Kagan, 2025). In education, AI literacy is needed to use and adapt virtual patient simulations, adaptive learning platforms, and intelligent tutoring systems that create tailored learning experiences. AI literacy is needed to develop institutional policies that both support AI integration in education and practice, academic integrity in learning, and ethical practice. Embedding digital literacy in nursing education prepares students for real-world healthcare environments.

Critical Thinking and Ethical Practice Beyond digital literacy, the introduction of AI and other technologies highlights the need to develop and enhance critical thinking, clinical reasoning and judgement, and ethical and humanistic practice. Recognizing the limits of technology, discovering or awareness of potential application of biases, and considering data and results within a nurses' clinical expertise and ethical framework are key elements to using AI. There are many opportunities for AI to be used in nursing education to elevate reflective practice and critical thinking skills. The application of ethical frameworks embedded in professional standards related to inclusion, data privacy and protection serve as an important guide as AI generated "solutions" are proposed. The use of AI in the educational setting also provides an opportunity to elevate academic integrity.

Cultivating Innovation and Leadership in Technology Use Finally, nurses and nurse educators should embrace their role as innovators and developers in the use and design of AI technology. Moving from adaptive and passive users to active designers and leaders is needed. Applying elements of design thinking: empathy—incorporating the perspective of learners and patients, defining goals, freedom to ideate and manage possible uses of AI, prototyping and testing are key strategies to be used in clinical and teaching contexts to promote optimal outcomes and essential learning. Importantly, integrating design thinking into education will serve nurses well in the practice setting.

The integration of AI into healthcare and nursing education presents both transformative opportunities and critical challenges. Building on nursing's primary focus of individuals and families, a strong ethical foundation, and innovative mind-set, nurses are well-positioned to lead AI advances in education and practice. By fostering digital literacy, and applying ethical frameworks and innovative practice, educators and practitioners can harness AI to enhance learning, improve patient care, and uphold professional standards. The future of nursing lies not just in adapting to technology, but in actively shaping its use to support equitable, safe, and human-centered practice.

Afterward

Angela Frederick Amar

When I think about artificial intelligence in nursing, I don't start with code. I start with people.

The power and promise of technology is dazzling. It's easy to get distracted by the glittering possibilities—so much that we focus on what AI can do, and forget to ask what people need.

This book provides a comprehensive, strategic roadmap for navigating the use of artificial intelligence in nursing education and practice. It explores the impacts, applications, and ethical challenges of AI in healthcare, and the critical role educators play in shaping its use as they train the next generation of nurse leaders.

At best, AI is an amplifier. It can magnify insight, scale simulation, support just-in-time learning, and expose risk earlier in care settings, but it can also magnify inequities, reproduce bias, and blur accountability.

This guide doesn't just offer just tools and frameworks for today. It highlights the questions we should ask—over and over and over again—as technology and the profession evolve. Among them: Who benefits? Who is excluded? What are we giving up in the name of efficiency and convenience? Are we seeing patients as people or data points? What should never be automated?

Are we chasing the shiny thing, or the right thing?

Nurses are the backbone of healthcare, and it's vital that we drive the conversation about AI in healthcare—when to use it, and when not to. We must teach students to integrate AI insights with clinical judgment, using technology to enhance, not replace, compassionate care.

As we move into this uncharted future, it is important that nurses have a seat at the tables of discovery and decisions. We must lead in making sure that artificial intelligence is used to benefit patients and patient care while being informed by nurses who provide much of the care. The future will bring even more intelligent and predictive systems. However, will they also help make nurses better? Will they increase the humanity of healthcare or cause nurses to interact more with systems

A. F. Amar
College of Nursing, New York University Rory Meyers College, New York, NY, USA
e-mail: angela.amar@nyu.edu

than with patients? Nurses must work to continually assess and align the values, codes, and practice with the technological advances of artificial intelligence.

As nurse educators, administrators, clinicians and policymakers, we have a duty to learn how to thrive at the intersection of progress and people's needs—and lead the way for the rest of the healthcare profession.

GPSR Compliance
The European Union's (EU) General Product Safety Regulation (GPSR) is a set
of rules that requires consumer products to be safe and our obligations to
ensure this.

If you have any concerns about our products, you can contact us on

ProductSafety@springernature.com

In case Publisher is established outside the EU, the EU authorized
representative is:

Springer Nature Customer Service Center GmbH
Europaplatz 3
69115 Heidelberg, Germany

www.ingramcontent.com/pod-product-compliance
Ingram Content Group UK Ltd.
Pitfield, Milton Keynes, MK11 3LW, UK
UKHW021826270126
467390UK00005B/52